# MIDNIGHT SHIFT

## A DR ELIZABETH BROOKS MYSTERY

LINDA RAWLINS

# MIDNIGHT SHIFT

Midnight Shift
A Dr Elizabeth Brooks Mystery

By Linda Rawlins



E-Book: 978-0-9600549-1-6
Paperback: 978-0-9600549-0-9

Discover other titles by Linda Rawlins at
**www.lindarawlins.com**

# ACKNOWLEDGMENTS

It takes an author to write a book but it takes a village to polish a novel. I sincerely want to thank everyone who has helped me with Midnight Shift.

My first circle of readers – Joe Liotti, Joyce Rawlins, Krista O'Neill, Sandi Chapin, Anita Uotinen– your editing tips, feedback and encouragement were vital to this book!

To everyone including Cathy Howe Stewart and Lisa Doster for cover feedback!

The staff of Riverbench Publishing – Matt Liotti, Ashley Liotti, Krista O'Neill – you are amazing with all you do.

To Joe – for all your support – from coffee to questions!!

To all my readers, librarians and booksellers, your friendship, encouragement and feedback spurs me on! Thank you!

Sweet Dreams!

*Dedicated to*

*Anita and Sandi*

*for sharing the journey from the beginning.*

*Thank You!*

# CHAPTER 1

"We've got blood."

"Dammit. What the hell is bleeding? Suction. I will not lose this patient." The rest of the team tensed palpably as the surgeon pulled down the drape and turned to the resident. "Get in here and clear the field."

She stepped back allowing the resident better access. He worked quickly to rid the wound of the rapidly spreading, red blood stain. Precious seconds later, he moved aside to allow the surgeon to return.

She continued to work, removing diseased tissue and repairing damage.

"His pressure is dropping, I'm pushing fluids now." Standing up, the anesthesiologist hung an extra IV bag.

"Damn, we're almost done. Let's tie the last bleeder and get out of here." Beads of sweat lined the surgeon's forehead as she worked to make sure all was taken care of. After a few moments, she was satisfied the bleeding was staunched in the patient's abdomen and called the resident to her side to help close the fat and muscle layers. Once he was ready, she turned to the OR nurse. "What about the sponge count? Is everything correct?"

"Everything is accounted for," the nurse said as she nodded at the team.

"Great, then let's finish this." She gestured to the resident and together they pulled the patient's skin together. The surgeon held while the resident stapled.

She turned to the anesthesiologist. "How's he doing?" Watching the monitors, she took in the patient's vital signs while waiting for an answer.

"Pressure is coming up," the anesthesiologist said as he adjusted the various gasses he was using to keep the patient sedated. "His heart rhythm looks good, we should be fine."

Dr. Elizabeth Brooks wasn't happy and stepped back to watch the patient fully stabilize. It should have been a simple cholecystectomy. She had promised the patient removing a gallbladder was one of the most common operations performed. What the hell happened?

Once the wound was dressed and surgical drapes adjusted, the surgical team came together to transfer the patient to the gurney. They lined up side by side and grabbed the edge of the rolled drape. On a defined count, they carefully slid the patient off the surgical table. The surgeon watched for a few more minutes as the anesthesiologist detached his equipment so the patient could be mobilized to the surgical intensive care unit.

As the transport team collected everything they needed, Dr. Brooks mentally reviewed what she wanted to document. She had read the pre-op notes, looked over the consents, double checked the CT scans, read the history and physical, reviewed the EKG and lab results, and carefully scanned the medication and allergy lists. The team held two time outs to make sure they knew what they were doing to whom before they started. She was sure nothing was missed.

She watched as the gurney rolled out of the operating suite, then properly disposed of her gown, gloves, and surgical hair net. Walking through the locker room, she changed into a clean set of blue scrubs and donned her hospital issued white lab coat. She immediately sat in front of the computer to get her orders in as quickly as possible.

Waiting for the software to open, she rehashed the procedure over and over. Mr. Byron was stable. The surgery ended well, but what the hell happened? Dr. Brooks spent the next forty minutes completing her documentation. The case was officially over but for some reason, she still had a knot in her stomach.

# CHAPTER 2

Dr. Elizabeth Brooks walked down the hallway of the hospital toward the surgical ICU. She had been on staff for five years and had plenty of experience, but lately her assigned cases were more difficult. Human Anatomy and Physiology had not changed in hundreds of years, but recently the patients were bleeding or bursting vessels that should have been strong and healthy.

"Hey, you got time for coffee?"

Elizabeth looked up to see her good friend, Caitlyn O'Rourke, pacing her in the hall. "I hate to break your deep brooding, but you look like you need a strong cup of coffee and I hear they have fresh vanilla almond in the café today."

Elizabeth laughed. "Do I look that bad?"

Caitlyn raised an eyebrow in reproach. "You actually have to ask me that? If you were on a busy street, you could have walked straight into a bus without noticing it coming."

"I think I would have noticed a bus," Elizabeth said as they reached the end of the hallway and turned into the cafeteria. The two women busied themselves picking up heavy coffee mugs and filling them with flavored coffee and cream. "Let's go sit in the physician's area. There's no one in there at the moment."

Caitlyn added pastry to her tray and picked it up. Walking to the room, she said, "It's good to be friends with the boss. The chairs are less sticky and the tables are clean."

Elizabeth laughed once again. "You don't like the physician area?"

"What's not to like? They take a part of the cafeteria, surround it with fake palm trees and clean it more often."

Shaking her head, Elizabeth picked a table and sat down. She sipped at her coffee and waited for Caitlyn to settle.

"What's wrong with you?" Caitlyn asked. "You look like you have the weight of the world on your shoulders."

Elizabeth shook her head. "I just had a bad case and it bothers the hell out of me." She looked at Caitlyn. "The patient is fine, but it should have been a routine case and it went sideways. This is the third one. I don't know why it's happening."

Caitlyn picked up her pastry and offered it to Elizabeth.

"No thanks, I'm not particularly hungry right now."

Taking a bite, Caitlyn asked, "So what do you think went wrong?"

Elizabeth paused for a moment. "This is the third case where a patient bled when he shouldn't have. It doesn't make sense. I've spent extra time looking over the med lists, making sure there's no blood thinner involved and the patient still bleeds more than they should. I'm starting to get paranoid."

"Has anyone else in the department had a problem?" Caitlyn asked.

"Not that I've heard of." Elizabeth took another sip of coffee and shook her head. "I'll have to bring it up to the department head. Maybe present the case at surgical rounds and see if anyone else has had something similar happen."

"Sounds like a plan," Caitlyn said as she popped the last bite of pastry in her mouth. She washed it down with a gulp of coffee. "Unfortunately, Dr. Pruitt will be an ass about it just because you brought it to his attention. Are you sure you want to do that?"

"I don't know. I'll have to think about it." Elizabeth was quiet for a minute, then turned to her friend. "So what have you been up to?"

"They stuck me in Intensive Care for the next week. I hate being a float nurse. I'm calling your office manager and telling him I want my old job back."

"Oh boy, I can only imagine the two of us working together again. You'd have to use your indoor voice." Elizabeth chuckled.

Caitlyn smirked. "I do what I have to do." She dusted off her hands and looked up. "What's the name of your patient? I'll keep a good eye on him."

"I'd appreciate that. His name is Randall Byron. He's a great guy. I feel bad because he was so anxious about the whole thing. I assured him it was a common surgery, but now he's had a complication."

"Well, he'll be fine," Caitlyn said. She took a few minutes to look at Elizabeth. "Have you been sleeping?"

Elizabeth sighed and shook her head. "You know I haven't slept well in the last twenty-five years."

"Are you taking your medication?"

It was Elizabeth's turn to grimace as she looked around the area. "I take it occasionally, but not before I have a case. I don't want a hang-over effect from medication. And, by the way, no one else knows about my meds or problem so I'd appreciate you keeping your voice down. You're sworn to confidentiality."

"I know, I've never had a HIPPA breach and I'm not going to start now. I wouldn't even know about it if you hadn't slept on my couch for a week after you broke up with that jerk you were dating."

"That was a definite emergency and I appreciate you being such a good friend. I had nowhere else to stay."

"Yes, I understand that and I know you were emotionally strained but having stress dreams which morph into PTSD dreams can be a struggle for yourself and those who can hear you in the surrounding area. Maybe you should go back to the doctor?"

Elizabeth stood up and brushed off her white jacket. "I'm going to get a coffee to go. How about you join me?"

"If I must," Caitlyn said as she sighed, picked up her empty coffee mug and followed Elizabeth across the café.

# CHAPTER 3

Elizabeth and Caitlyn walked to the surgical ICU together. When they reached the unit, Caitlyn swiped in and went off to get her assignment. Elizabeth made her way to the nursing station and started gathering post-op information on her patient. She opened his chart to check his vitals as well as any reports of pain or complications. Noting that all remained stable, Elizabeth entered his cubicle to visit. His eyes were closed and he lay unmoving on the pillow. Elizabeth noted his skin was gray and cool to touch as she softly called his name several times without a response. Looking at his chest, she felt a flurry of anxiety when she didn't notice any rise or fall. Her head snapped to the monitor which showed a slow rhythm. Without realizing, she held his wrist in her hand and began to squeeze as she watched the monitors. When he let out a loud snore, she jumped and gulped air as her own heart banged in her chest.

Elizabeth let go of Mr. Byron's wrist and backed away from the bed. She sat in the chair for a moment as a slight headache pressured her temple. When the symptoms resolved, she stood up and went back to the bedside. Nervously, she pulled down the blanket to check the abdominal dressing. She dreaded finding the bandage soiled but when she examined the area, she found nothing but dry, clean, white bandages. No sign of blood or excessive bleeding. "Thank you, Lord," she whispered to herself as she pulled the blankets back up and tucked him in. She adjusted the stethoscope hanging around her neck and stood quietly for a moment.

When she turned to leave, she found Caitlyn standing at the doorway. "Find anything I need to worry about under there?"

Elizabeth shook her head. "Nope, everything is clean and dry. I think he's still sedated from the procedure."

"Excellent, now get out and let me do my job." Caitlyn grabbed her arm as Elizabeth started to pass by. "Heads up, pissant Pruitt is at the nurse's station making someone's life miserable and I don't mean a patient."

"Thanks for the warning," Elizabeth said with a frown. "I have to go document, but if I'm lucky, he's already moved on."

Elizabeth left the ICU cubicle, saw Dr. Pruitt was still at the nurse's station, and headed toward the exit. She planned to document on Mr. Byron's chart but considering she could access her computer from her office, she decided to get out of the hospital as soon as possible. She quickly walked toward the sliding glass doors when a male voice boomed out to get her attention.

"Dr. Brooks, wait a moment, please," Dr. Pruitt commanded.

After silently cursing in her head, she stopped, drew up to her full height and turned around to face the department chief. "Yes, good morning, Dr. Pruitt. How can I help you?"

"Can I have a private moment?" Dr. Pruitt gestured toward a small alcove in the hospital hall. Unfortunately, when they arrived near the alcove, he barely lowered his voice. "I wanted to let you know your last case has been scheduled for discussion in front of the hospital medical board."

Elizabeth stiffened at his words which she imagined gave him perverse pleasure to deliver. "Oh, really? Why is that?"

Pruitt's smile was cruel. "As you know there has been concern about your surgical acumen. Besides being a major concern for the quality of our service, your failed cases are impacting the mortality rate and quality data of our department, as well as the hospital in general."

Feelings of rage engulfed Elizabeth. So much for discussing the abnormalities with the department. "The outcome of those cases had nothing to do with my surgical *acumen.*" She practically spit the words back at him. "The two patient deaths were very sad and unfortunate but had nothing to do with surgical technique during the procedure."

Pruitt cleared his throat. "The department has yet to meet with you to discuss the Burdette case. I just rounded on my patients in the unit and I heard the nurses talking. Am I to understand you've had another issue in surgery today?"

Elizabeth took a moment, shoved her fists into the pockets of her white coat and cleared her throat.

"As a matter of fact, I was planning to speak with you about that patient."

"That's very interesting because it appeared you were running out of the Surgical ICU. I assume you must have noticed my presence when you came out of the patient's cubicle."

"Dr. Pruitt, I assure you I was planning on speaking to you and addressing the department about this patient. The procedure went well from the standpoint of technique. Unfortunately, near the end, the patient started to bleed for unknown reasons. We were not working in the area which bled, so there could not have been a surgical misstep. In all honesty, I was wondering if there could be another problem."

"That's preposterous, Dr. Brooks. There have been no other problems in this surgical department."

"Do you know that as fact?" Elizabeth questioned. "Have you discussed unsuspected bleeding with the entire department? Have you audited cases? Perhaps some of the staff members are not comfortable coming forth to speak with you." She finished her statement with a small, sweet smile. The color of Dr. Pruitt's face zoomed past red to purple in a quick second.

"Your insubordination is astounding, Dr. Brooks. I assure you this conversation will be brought to higher levels within our hospital." Dr.

Pruitt turned around and strode down the hall, past the elevator and banged the door on his way through the stairway exit.

Elizabeth shook her head and made her way to the locker room to change out of her blues. When she was done, she slowly brushed her hair and with a deep sigh walked out of the hospital.

# CHAPTER 4

Sitting at the desk in her office, Elizabeth sipped another cup of decaffeinated coffee. She hated Monday mornings. Glancing at her schedule, she savored the last few moments of peace and quiet she would have all day. As a busy surgeon, who also practiced a small amount of office medicine, she kept a hectic schedule. When the office released the answering service, the phone would start ringing, all four lines glowing at once. She'd receive the weekend report from the local hospitals, nursing home, and the covering doctor. She'd also receive messages from the patients who tolerated their symptoms over the weekend.

Elizabeth finished her coffee, examined her schedule and headed toward the exam rooms. Out of the corner of her eye, she saw Ruth running toward her with a handful of messages that just couldn't wait. Ruth was in her late 50's, with gray streaked, dark hair, twisted into a tight bun. Ruth was anxious about getting everything done in a precise manner on a daily basis.

Elizabeth turned toward Ruth and tried to smile when Ruth bombarded her with the list of patients who had called for appointments, referrals, refills, test results or wanted their surgical site checked.

"I'm sorry, Dr. Brooks," Ruth said as she shook her head. "The message book is filling up and I don't know what to do with these patients. Heather already started with the first patient and Molly has a line at the registration window. How do you want me to handle these messages?"

Elizabeth took a deep breath. "As usual, one by one."

Ruth handed the pile to Elizabeth who quickly flipped through them making sure there was no bad news from the hospital. When she was done, she handed them back to Ruth.

"Please put them on my message board and I'll triage them in-between patients."

Just then, Heather emerged from the first exam room and put a chart in the plastic bin on the door. She brushed by Elizabeth and whispered, "Good luck with this one," and tilted her head toward the exam room. Heather had worked with Elizabeth for four years now. She was a good RN. She helped organize the patient flow through the office and served as Elizabeth's right and left hand throughout most of the day. More importantly, she kept Ruth calm. Elizabeth had hired Heather to replace Caitlyn, when she left for a higher paying position in the hospital.

"Heather, could you please look through these messages and help Ruth triage them on the communication board? I'll start working on them when I'm done with the first patient."

Heather grinned and nodded her head. "You're not going to be done with the first patient for awhile, so we'll start pulling the charts as well." Heather took Ruth by the arm and steered her back to the main reception area while Elizabeth approached the exam room. She lifted the chart from its rack and knocked on the door.

"Come in," snapped a male voice. Elizabeth slowly opened the door. On the table was an 87 year old gentleman, naked from the waist up. Elizabeth glanced at his chart as she stepped into the exam room.

"Excuse me, Mr. Martin?"

"Just call me, Lucky, ma'am."

"Okay, Lucky. Why are you half naked?"

"I figured that's what you needed me to do. If it's a problem, don't let the cranky doctor know."

"Lucky, I am the cranky doctor and it's not necessary."

Lucky's eyes opened wide as he noted his new doctor was a graceful blonde in her early thirties. She looked lean and strong, yet vulnerable.

"Lucky, I'm going to leave the exam room for a minute and you can put your shirt back on, for now. When I get back, I'd like to go over your history and physical, talk about your meds and then I'll do an exam."

"Thanks, Doc. That's not how they did it in the military."

"I'm sure, but you can relax now."

Elizabeth handed him his pile of clothes and left the exam room. She stood in the hall and visualized being on the beach. As she waited for him to get dressed, she glanced through the small paper chart. She'd review the rest of the electronic chart when she went back into the exam room.

Mr. John Martin, also known as Lucky, was a veteran of the Korean War. He suffered from diabetes, high blood pressure, high cholesterol, and prostate problems. He was asking for a screen for dementia. He took several medications and was trying to find a doctor closer to home. He appeared to have quite a sense of humor as well.

Elizabeth knocked on the door. "Mr. Martin, are you dressed?"

"Yes, doctor," he replied in an angelic tone.

Elizabeth opened the door to the exam room. Lucky was fully dressed and sitting in the chair by the wall. So far, so good. "Good morning, Mr. Martin. My name is Dr. Elizabeth Brooks. I am the physician. How are you today?"

"Same as I was ten minutes ago, but otherwise alright."

Elizabeth nodded and went on with the medical interview.

"Can you tell me what brought you here today?'

"Why, the senior bus, of course," replied Lucky.

Elizabeth couldn't help smiling in spite of herself. "Mr. Martin, Lucky, how can I help you?"

Lucky glanced at Elizabeth and his expression became more serious. "Look, Doc, I need someone who will sit and listen to me. The talk about town is that you care about your patients."

Elizabeth flinched inside at Lucky's mention of her reputation. She did care about her patients and she was very concerned about her reputation after she had two patients die in the last six months. Lucky continued to speak which brought her back to the present.

"I thought I'd see if you could be my doctor. I need someone good. I feel like crap lately, like a dead body who happens to be walking."

"Why do you say that?"

"Because nothing works anymore. I constantly have pain and I can't hold my urine. I'm embarrassed and suffering all the time. My old doctor just keeps giving me more pills. He says I shouldn't expect anything more because I'm old. His attitude is insulting besides the fact that I can't afford the pills."

Realizing Lucky's behavior was a major defense mechanism against some serious emotions, Elizabeth swiped to the first page of the electronic chart and said, "Let's look at some information and see what we can offer." Despite a rocky start to their appointment, Elizabeth already felt sorry for the codger. "Tell me more about your past medical history."

"Well, I've had sugar for the past four years. It's usually on the high side. If I take the pill, the sugar is better, but then I have stomach cramps and gas. I don't know if I can afford injections anymore. I'm also supposed to take medicine for my blood pressure and my cholesterol."

"Lucky, when was your last blood test?"

"I think last year sometime. I read in the senior magazines that diabetics are supposed to have a special blood test on a regular basis. It's hard for me to get to a lab or I'm too depressed to care. I know they're going to find something horrible someday."

Elizabeth nodded her head and typed on her keyboard. She purposely had special writing desks installed in her office so she could face her patient, document in the computer, and be able to hold a direct conversation while keeping her notes.

"Lucky, you mentioned prostate problems. Tell me more about that."

"It started about six years ago. I'd go to the bathroom and five minutes later I'd have to go back. I thought it was an infection so I went to a doctor. He said my prostate was big and I needed an operation. So I had the surgery. I don't have cancer, but I have trouble holding my urine."

"When was the last time you saw your urologist?"

Lucky's expression was dismissive. "Who knows? I'm not going back to that doctor anymore. He says he can't do anything else for me and gave me a coupon for diapers. Can you believe it? I was a sergeant in the Korean War and now I'm wearing diapers." He wiped a tear from the corner of his eye.

Elizabeth could see he was a proud man. "Will you tell me about your military experience?"

Lucky coughed and looked at her, his expression unreadable. "Doc, I was in North Korea. I was a sergeant on Heartbreak Ridge, back in the 50's. It was rainy, it was muddy. It was miserable . A lot of guys didn't make it back, but I did. I was in pretty poor shape, but I made it. That's how I got my nickname, Lucky. I shouldn't have made it, Doc, but I did."

"I'm happy you did, Lucky. I'm glad I've met you and thank you for serving."

"Thanks, Doc. I signed up because my family didn't have any money. I was pretty smart and eventually made it to Sergeant. We did okay, but Heartbreak Ridge was tough. You know, I still see the guys in my head. I dream about them, wake up crying and my heart is pounding. You have no idea how rough it was."

"Actually, I'm very familiar with dreams," Elizabeth said with a small smile.

Lucky shook his head. "I keep dreaming about legs lying on the ground. That's one thing I did in Korea. I retrieved every body part I found, so I could bring them home. There were times when I didn't know who the body part belonged to. It didn't matter. I had to get everything and send it home. I wouldn't have wanted to leave my legs in Korea if they got blown off. Now, some of my toes and fingertips are numb. I was told it was from the wet and cold, but one of the docs thinks it's from diabetes. They called it neuro something." Lucky made a fist with each hand. "They may be numb, but at least they're attached."

Elizabeth smiled. "Lucky, the condition is called peripheral neuropathy. You can get it for a number of reasons, but from having uncontrolled diabetes as well."

"Well, my toes were numb for a long time before I knew about the sugar."

Elizabeth nodded. She acknowledged how this man had suffered over the years. His behavior was just an act to cover the pain, loneliness and anxiety he had felt many times since being in Korea.

"Do you have family?" She asked.

Lucky shook his head. "No, I dated for awhile when I got back to the States but it's hard to have a relationship when your head is screwed up."

"What about your parents?"

"My dad died from a heart attack when he was 47. My mom died from, I don't know what," he said with a shrug. "She had the sugar too. She had her leg cut off and she died right after that." He hung his head for a moment. "I miss them. My mom was my world to me."

No wonder he was so attached to body parts. "You've been alone for a long time."

Lucky shrugged again. "I connected with my buddies on and off. A lot of us were messed up and either didn't marry or got divorced. We'd work as mechanics or do something close to what we did in the military. A lot of the guys have died. It hasn't been easy, Doc."

Elizabeth looked down at his electronic chart again. She felt strongly about patients who suffered in this world. There were many kinds of suffering and as much as she griped each day, she reminded herself she should be happy with life.

"Lucky," Elizabeth smiled and touched his hand. "Do you ever check your sugar with a glucometer?"

"Is that one of those little meter things?"

"Yes, you have to stick yourself with a pin and then you test the drop of blood to see what your sugar level is. Maybe, if we do a better job with your sugar, including some diet and exercise, we can make sure you don't lose any of your toes. What do you think?"

"I think that sounds great," Lucky said with a smile. "You know, Doc, you're okay. If I survived Korea, I can tolerate a little pin each day."

"Let's start with your diabetes and we can work on other things later." She squeezed his arm. "Use the pain medicine that you have. Is there anything else you're worried about?"

Lucky thought for a moment. "Yes, there's one more thing I wanted to ask you. Sometimes, I walk from one room into another and I can't remember what I wanted."

"That's normal for a lot of us depending on your sugar, or how much sleep you got the night before."

"Well, I don't want to wind up losing my mind. I heard there's a new supplement out there for people who can't remember things. What if I start that?"

"Do you know the name of the supplement?"

Lucky shook his head as he laughed. "No, I can't remember, Doc."

"Let's start with making sure your sugar is the best it can be and then we'll work on your other problems. That way, we'll know exactly what problems are related to what."

Lucky nodded. "Sounds good. I'm sorry I gave you a hard time. I guess once you learn to fight for everything you have, you're just afraid to stop."

Elizabeth smiled. "Come on, let's go to the lab, and draw some blood."

# CHAPTER 5

Reaching the end of office hours, Elizabeth was back at her desk. She had pushed off her heels and was rubbing the arches of her feet when Heather popped in. "How are you doing?"

Elizabeth laughed. "The usual. I'm tired and my feet hurt. I've been standing since I started the 5:00 a.m. surgical case this morning."

"Well, I hate to be the bearer of bad news, but you had one last patient in the waiting room. Apparently, Ruth added him several hours ago, but didn't put the patient's name on your tablet."

"Really?" Elizabeth's head tensed. She was tired and happy she had made it to the end of the patient portion of the day. There was still plenty of work to be done. Reviewing lab results, patient phone calls, notes to be completed and locked into the computer.

"I'm sorry. She didn't run it by me before she scheduled him and now he's in one of the exam rooms. A guy named Jake Wagner. He's here to have his blood pressure checked."

"Was it high?" Elizabeth asked. "If he just wants a screening, you can do that and he can come back for multiple readings."

"It was mildly elevated," Heather said.

"Why are you acting funny?" Elizabeth asked. "Is there something you're not telling me?"

Heather shook her head. "I don't know. I'm being silly, but I just have a weird vibe about this guy. He doesn't seem like a typical patient."

"Do we need to call the police?"

"Well, that's just it. He came into the exam room wearing a suit. I made him take his jacket off so I could check his blood pressure. He was hesitant, but he finally did and that's when I noticed he was wearing a gold shield."

"Oh, really?"

"Something's off, so I think you should go talk to the man yourself. Find out what his secondary agenda is."

Elizabeth took a deep breath and braced herself. "It's already been a bad day. I hope he's not going to make it worse."

Heather shrugged. "Only one way to find out, but I want to point out he is incredibly handsome. Dark hair, blue eyes and very attractive." She reached over the desk and handed Elizabeth the demographic paper chart. Elizabeth frowned, opened the folder and scanned the information.

*Mr. Jake Wagner, Age 34, Address - blank, Occupation - blank, PMH – Past medical history - blank, Chief complaint – headaches.*

"There's nothing in here. He didn't fill out the registration sheet."

"And there's my point," Heather said. "Go check it out."

Elizabeth's stomach clenched as she put her shoes on, got up from her desk and made her way to the exam room. She knocked on the door, waited a few seconds, and then entered. An attractive, muscular, well groomed man was standing across the room reading a chart attached to the wall.

"Mr. Wagner?"

"Yes, that's me." As he turned, she noted he was dressed in an expensive suit and had put his jacket back on.

Elizabeth nodded and extended her hand. "My name is Dr. Elizabeth Brooks. How can I help you today?"

Jake's chiseled chin dimpled when he smiled. He looked down for a moment and then back up at Elizabeth. "I wanted to meet you and hoped we could talk for a few minutes."

Elizabeth shifted, but did not smile. Her senses were on alert. "I'm afraid I don't understand, Mr. Wagner. Heather told me you were here for mild hypertension, but you make it sound like something else."

"I'll admit, my appointment was a ruse to make sure I was able to speak with you."

"I still don't understand what you're after."

Mr. Wagner moved his jacket to the side to reveal the gold badge on the waistband of his pants. "Let me reintroduce myself. I'm Detective Jake Wagner with the New Wales Police Department. I'm looking for some information on one of your patients."

Elizabeth didn't immediately respond. After a second, she said, "Then you already know I can't give you information unless you have the proper legal paperwork. Between patient-client confidentiality and HIPPA, I can't tell you anything. Why did you make an appointment? Why not just walk in and flash your badge?"

"Because I'm conducting a routine investigation and I purposely didn't want to upset you. How about if I talk and you listen?"

Elizabeth sat down on the office stool. "I guess I can do that, but don't expect me to answer anything."

"Deal," Jake said as he perched himself against the edge of the exam table. "I'm here investigating a gentleman by the name of Frank Burdette. I believe you know who he is."

Elizabeth's face flashed red. "I can neither confirm or deny he was my patient."

"You see, that's the key word right there, was."

Elizabeth shot to her feet. "What exactly are you implying?"

Jake stood up to calm her. "I'm not implying anything. I know the man is dead and I've read the coroner's report."

"Then you know he died of a ruptured aortic aneurysm. The surgery I performed had nothing to do with the aorta."

"Take it easy," Jake replied. "I'm not here about the surgery. I was asked to investigate the guy long before he had surgery. It seems there was some concern about his work performance. He was the financial officer for a start up company. There were some irregularities with their books and we were asked to investigate. At first he denied everything, but then started evading us whenever we showed up to meet with him. At one point, we brought him in for questioning and pressed him with some of the information we had. He didn't want to go down for the company so he agreed to an exchange of information for a suspended sentence, but he was afraid for his life if he was found out. He said he needed to get something for us. A journal or maybe a second set of books. Who knows? Anyway, we set a date to meet with him and have a complete debriefing, brought the FBI in as well, and the guy baled. He left a message that he had an important doctor's appointment and couldn't meet. When we showed up at his home with the arrest warrant, we found out he was dead." Jake paced the room as he stroked his chin. He faced Elizabeth and spread his hands. "So now you see my dilemma. I'm here to check that his health, his appointment, and even his surgery and subsequent death are all just coincidental."

"Well, whatever it is, it had nothing to do with my surgical technique. I had no knowledge of anything regarding his company. Furthermore, if you read the autopsy report, you can see the man had some real disease. The complications were simply that, complications." Elizabeth stopped and stared for a moment as awareness crept in. "It's bad enough my department chief is claiming bad technique, but I hope you aren't implying I was involved or would purposely cause a fatal complication?" Elizabeth waited a few seconds. "Are you?"

Jake shook his head. "No, absolutely not. We're simply looking into the facts."

Elizabeth was now fully annoyed. She raised her voice as she pointed at him. "The fact is the man came to this office for health reasons. I didn't know him personally or anyone associated with him. He died of unexpected complications in post-op which still can't be explained, but I wasn't there at the time as I was in the OR working on another case." Elizabeth took a breath. "I think you should leave immediately or I will call my attorney and your chief and have you reprimanded for harassment." She opened the door and gestured for him to leave. Jake looked up and noticed Heather arrive at the door. Heather's eyes flicked back and forth between Elizabeth and Jake Wagner. Elizabeth handed her the chart and said, "Please escort Mr. Wagner to the front door and make sure he pays his copay before he leaves."

# CHAPTER 6

Elizabeth was still fuming when she got home. She went to the fridge and pulled out a cold bottle of Merlot. Pouring a glass she sipped the wine while she checked her mail, email and texts. Before she left the office, she called the Surgical Intensive Care Unit to make sure Mr. Byron was stable. Caitlyn answered the phone and gave an efficient report. He hadn't been assigned to her for the day, but when Caitlyn went on shift, she made arrangements to switch him to her caseload for one of her other patients. Caitlyn had checked on his vitals and pain every hour. He remained a bit groggy from the anesthesia, but was making small progress to date. Since Caitlyn had pulled a twelve hour shift, she told Elizabeth to calm down and relax for the night while she kept watch.

Elizabeth sat at her kitchen table and pulled her iPad close to her while she waited for a frozen dinner to heat in the microwave. She finished her first glass of wine and poured a second as she waited for the iPad to fully open. After taking a sip, the bell sounded the completion of her microwave dinner which she pulled from the oven and placed on the table to cool.

After another sip of wine, she went back to her iPad and typed Jake Wagner in the search bar. She knew she wasn't supposed to search names and prayed that someone wasn't monitoring or checking her history, but she was steamed. Within a few seconds, images of Detective Jake Wagner appeared on her screen. The guy was solid and had only become more handsome with age.

She read his history with the New Wales Police Department. He had been working in the department for approximately ten years. As she continued to peruse the internet, she learned he had several accommodations for his police work. His promotions were listed with a photo celebrating each event.

Elizabeth shook her head and turned off her iPad. She pulled the cooled dinner near her place at the table and picked at it with her utensils. She sipped her wine and thought about what she read. He was a handsome detective. There was no mention of a wife or children but she supposed that was intentional so family would not become a target of angry felons he had helped capture. He hadn't been wearing a ring but that didn't mean he wasn't married or almost divorced with crippling child support. Perhaps he had a bevy of illegitimate children.

Elizabeth picked up her glass and finished the wine. She laughed while tears formed in her eyes and then acknowledged how silly she was acting. His words had surprised and frightened her to the point she became angry when she realized he was considering she could have been a part of or at fault for Frank Burdette's death. She worked so hard to advance her career to where it was today, just to have it ripped to shreds in months.

Growing up on the East Coast, Elizabeth was lucky to have attended medical school nearby. When Match day came along, she prayed and wished on every star that she would be paired with a medical residency near home. Her prayers were answered when she was chosen to work at a hospital in New Wales. It was a large, urban facility whose goal was to achieve the highest quality ratings possible. New Wales was a densely populated town. Near enough to a city to enjoy the excitement of bright lights but far enough to be away from the problems of parking and over-priced living. Elizabeth loved New Wales. Her parents lived at the Jersey Shore which was the perfect place to visit when she wanted to seek solace by the ocean, but far enough to maintain her privacy, especially when her demons came to town. Elizabeth poured a little more wine. Life had been busy but relatively happy for her in New Wales until things started happening six months prior.

After rinsing her dishes and glass, Elizabeth made her way to the bedroom. She was exhausted from a combination of the wine and the aggravation of the day, but dreaded going to sleep when she was stressed. She hoped the wine would sedate her enough to help her sleep through the night without her medication.

She changed, got into bed and placed her head on the cool pillow. She fell asleep almost instantly, but within 45 minutes, she began to moan in her sleep. Her body tossed and turned as images flew across her mind.

*THE ROOM WAS DARK, she couldn't see the furniture but she knew it was there. She looked around the room, but didn't recognize the place. It wasn't her childhood home but somehow she felt connected as if she had visited many, many years ago. Elizabeth slowly walked toward the only source of light in the room. A window overlooking the sidewalk below. It was dark, but she couldn't pin the time. There, in the streetlight, she saw a teenage girl kneel to the pavement with her arms extended. A happy dog jumped into her arms, tail wagging. The girl hugged the dog to her chest, a smile on her face. Immediately, sadness poured from Elizabeth's mind. The girl's youth and the dog represented the passage of time, happier days gone by and a loss of innocence. She was grieving in her sleep.*

ALTHOUGH SHE WAS ASLEEP, Elizabeth could hear herself moan and cry out. She woke up sobbing and feeling incredibly sad. She wasn't sure what bothered her more, having the dreams return or the realization she might be losing control.

# CHAPTER 7

Blue skies greeted Elizabeth when she woke the next morning. Initially, she hadn't been able to get back to sleep for several hours, but then was exhausted enough to finally drop off. She had probably gotten four hours of sleep if she added it all together. Thank goodness, she wasn't scheduled for surgery today.

Elizabeth crawled out of bed and padded into the kitchen to start a strong pot of coffee. She spied the near empty wine bottle and hesitated before she dumped the rest of the contents into the sink. She hadn't come home and had alcohol in years, but the stress was beginning to overwhelm her. She had hoped the wine would help her sleep but now she wondered if it exacerbated her dreams. The abandonment of her healthy lifestyle program due to stress in the last six months hadn't help.

She checked her morning messages and email as she gulped a cup of coffee and dressed for the day. She purposely arranged her schedule to have an easier day after performing surgery. The varied schedule allowed her to spend more time dealing with post-op patients and time to rest so she wouldn't be exhausted by the end of the week.

Pouring another cup of coffee into her travel thermos, she grabbed her belongings and left for the hospital. While she drove, she couldn't help reviewing the events of the prior day, especially her meeting with Detective Jake Wagner. Elizabeth didn't doubt the patient could have been involved in illicit activity. Probably a good percent of her patients were involved in something illegal. She could only control the things for which she was responsible, such as diagnosing disease, prescribing narcotics and being a good surgeon. Beyond that, their private life was just that, private and as long as they didn't ask for anything illegal, immoral or criminal, she treated their problems and moved on.

Elizabeth parked the car and made her way inside the hospital. She stopped at the locker room near the surgery suite and locked up her personal belongings. Carrying her coffee, she made her way to the surgical ICU.

She stopped at the main desk to check on any last minute labs or reports that hadn't made it to the computer yet. She asked for the nurse assigned to Randall Byron and indicated she would wait for her at the patient's bedside. Walking toward his cubicle, she was surprised to find Caitlyn in his room.

"What are you doing here? I thought you pulled twelve hours yesterday," Elizabeth said as she walked over to the monitors and took in the readings.

Caitlyn finished tucking in the blankets. "I did but then someone called out and they begged me to come back. Normally I'd tell them to buzz off, but I took the shift thinking I could get more info on your patient."

Elizabeth turned to look at her. "Thank you, Caitlyn. I appreciate you keeping a close eye on him. How's he doing?"

"So-so," Caitlyn said as she shrugged. "Listen, I've got a coffee break coming up. Why don't you finish your exam and then we can grab a cup together."

Elizabeth realized Caitlyn didn't want to speak in front of the patient and wanted to share something, so she readily agreed.

"I'll meet you at the desk in a moment. If they tell you I was looking for you, let them know you found me."

"You've got it," Caitlyn said as she pushed the curtain aside and left the cubicle.

Elizabeth turned back to Mr. Byron and gently called his name. "Hello, it's Dr. Brooks. How are you today?"

The patient grunted and tried to stir. "Mr. Byron, can you hear me? Are you having any pain?" Elizabeth tensed as she realized he should be more active than he currently was. She had performed a common surgery on his gallbladder. Most patients who had this type of surgery were discharged by now, but her patient appeared lethargic and confused. She gently pulled down the blankets and examined his belly. The surgical site was clean and dry. Caitlyn had done a great job with the dressing, but the patient should have been more alert. Elizabeth would question Caitlyn about the amount of pain medication he was taking when they had coffee. Mr. Byron had always been stoic so she would be surprised if he had requested extra medication. Taking a last look at the monitors, she pulled the blankets up and left the room.

Elizabeth walked toward the nurse's desk and caught Caitlyn's eye. She tilted her head toward the exit and both made their way out of the ICU without connecting in front of the rest of the staff. They came together in the hall and made their way toward the café.

"I'm glad I caught up with you," Caitlyn said as she pulled her blue scrub jacket around her body.

"Normally I would agree, but in this case, you have me asking why," Elizabeth said with a frown. They entered the café and both went to the coffee counter. They quietly grabbed cups, poured coffee and fixed it to their taste, before finding a seat in a private part of the room.

"Alright, enough already. Spit it out, what's going on? Is it about Mr. Byron?"

Caitlyn shook her head as she stared at her coffee. "Yes and no. First, Mr. Byron is just not where he should be after having his gallbladder out."

"Tell me about it," Elizabeth said. "What's going on? Can you pinpoint anything?"

Caitlyn looked up at Elizabeth. "I can't. He's just too lethargic. His blood pressure is lower than it should be and his repeat lab shows he's anemic."

"His surgical site looked clean and dry," Elizabeth said. "I checked it when I was in the cubicle just now. You place a mean bandage."

Caitlyn laughed. "Thanks. The entire abdomen looks great. His belly is soft, no bruising and no discharge, but he's just not responding."

"Shit," Elizabeth said softly as she looked at her friend. She picked up her coffee and noticed her hand was shaking slightly.

Caitlyn reached out and placed her hand on Elizabeth's arm. Elizabeth looked at her friend to find a smile plastered over a pity face. "What? What's wrong now?"

Caitlyn shook her head and teared slightly as she looked at Elizabeth. "I've fought with myself all day whether to tell you this."

Elizabeth put her coffee down. "Well, now you have to, so get to it."

"Pissant Pruitt was in the ICU with the administrator today."

"And?"

"First and foremost, they're a pair of asshats. Secondly, they shouldn't be discussing any of their thoughts in front of the staff, but it bears repeating that they're asshats."

"What were they discussing? I'm assuming it was me," Elizabeth said as she picked her coffee up again.

Caitlyn nodded. "Yes, they scoured Mr. Byron's chart and went to examine him. As we just said there was nothing specific going on so they couldn't suggest any change in the orders. As a matter of fact, the administrator supported you and said as much."

"Good, but.."

"Then Pruitt brings up the death of Frank Burdette and of course, the death of Connie Arturo."

"He is an ass," Elizabeth said with a shake of the head. "He's on a mission."

"Exactly. He was suggesting, very loudly I might add, that not only should you be called out on these cases in front of the executive board, but he wants you to lose your privileges permanently."

Elizabeth struggled to control her emotions as she felt the rage building inside. Her face turned red and she needed to breathe through her nose. "He keeps bringing up Burdette's case, but they've looked at the autopsy. He died from a ruptured aortic aneurysm which was nowhere near the surgical site. They reviewed the pre-op lab, scans and meds. There was nothing on pre-op to suggest he had a dangerous aneurysm. It's all rather odd. Then, the bastard tried to claim that I had possibly caused an aneurysm by leaning on my patient's abdomen during surgery. That's ridiculous and he wasn't able to fabricate anything else to challenge my technique."

Elizabeth took a deep breath and Caitlyn rubbed her arm. Swallowing, Elizabeth continued. "In addition, the fact that I won accolades over him for having such precise technique is the reason his ego is bruised. I don't know what the hell is going on lately, but it's not about my surgical prowess."

Caitlyn smiled. "You go, girl. Fight that blowhard. He's been terrorizing the medical staff far too long in this hospital."

"He can call me before the board, but I'll have my attorney at my side. They can present whatever proof they have and then finish the discussion in court as far as I'm concerned. I can't believe I have to go through this harassment."

"Amen to that," Caitlyn said as she looked at her watch. "I'm glad I decided to give you the head's up, but I'd better get back to the ICU to make sure Mr. Byron sticks around long enough to get discharged out the front door."

Elizabeth laughed. "Thank you for believing in me."

"You've got it, boss. I used to work in your office. I've seen you in action so it's not very hard to believe in your dedication. However, if I'm ever in need of removal of an organ or two, I expect you to do it for free."

Caitlyn realized it was nice to hear her friend laugh again as she ran out of the café to get back to work.

# CHAPTER 8

Jake stood at the scarred wooden desk in the squad room and looked through some of the papers stacked there. He wore another classic suit. His hand was on his hip, pushing back his jacket edge, revealing his gleaming badge from it's position on his waistband.

"Find anything?" His partner, Alex Houghton asked.

"I haven't had time to go through it all yet," Jake said. "But I'm telling you, the good doctor is going to be the key to this mystery."

Alex balled up the paper his lunch had arrived in and tossed it at Jake's head. "Are you sure your interest is confined to the vic?"

Jake pulled out an old chair and sat down. "Stick it, Alex. Finish your food, wash the jelly off your hands. Go get some steps."

Alex got up, flipped Jake the bird, and walked past several desks piled with papers as other detectives worked their cases.

Laughing, Jake turned back to his paperwork and flipped through the stack. They had received several calls about Frank Burdette and were in the middle of their investigation when he died. They would have easily classified it as a homicide except he had died in the hospital from a surgical complication. It was called a large vessel disorder. Something wasn't right about that as the arterial abnormality should have showed up on the pre-op CT scan according to Jake's sources. Jake admitted that he knew next to nothing about medicine. He was lucky if he got a band-aid to stick in the right direction after a cut, but the doctor would know. If she wasn't directly involved, she would be able to tell him where to look. Jake also wanted to know how someone could alter or create fake medical records in an electronic medical records system.

Alex returned from the bathroom and made it a point to hold his hands out in front of Jake. "What's your next move, Slayer?" Jake earned his nickname years ago after wearing nothing but fine suits to work. The ladies who worked in the department would go out of their way to visit his desk with food, innocently leaving their phone numbers with the dishes. The rest of the division didn't receive any attention, but they ate a lot of cake and for that they were grateful.

"As much as I hate to do it, I'm going to have to get my blood pressure rechecked," Jake sighed. "Sooner or later, she'll have to talk to me."

"Why did she feel so threatened the last time?"

"I don't know. Probably some jerk trying to lay this whole mess at her feet. Who knows?"

"Were you able to connect her to Frank anytime before we got the tip?" Alex asked as he grabbed a file.

Jake shook his head. "Nope, nothing. I combed his phone records, credit cards and whatever I could get my hands on in relation to his activities. No one recognized the Doc's photo. The guy didn't have credit card charges to hotel rooms or fancy restaurants. If anything, he was running into some big money problems. No, something else was going on, but I'll be damned if I can put my finger on it, yet." Jake tossed a file onto the desk and leaned back in his chair.

"Yeah, but what about the other death?" Alex asked, holding up a photograph.

"That's the strange thing. We know Frank and Connie knew each other but we can't tie either one to the doctor. Yet, both died by the doctor's hand within a few months of each other. We have a coroner's report for each one verifying they were absolutely dead and didn't skip the country. Very, very, strange."

"Were they having an affair?" Alex asked.

"Who? Frank and Connie? Or Frank and the doctor? Or Connie and the doctor for that matter? Not sure about any of that," Jake answered as he sat up straight in the chair. He grabbed his keys, adjusted his suit coat and looked at Alex. "C'mon, let's go."

"Where?"

"I made an appointment to talk with Connie's husband. Let's see if we can shake some trees."

"You got that right," Alex said as he slammed his desk drawer, stood and followed Jake out the door.

# CHAPTER 9

Elizabeth finished her coffee and left the café. She made her way to the medical records department to sign a few documents that had been transcribed and left in her folder. She always attended to her medical records immediately and precisely. She didn't want to wait any longer than necessary to ensure she had accurate details in her dictation. That's why she was dumbfounded when Frank Burdette died from the aortic aneurysm. She had gone over his CT scan with a fine tooth comb. She had read and reread the radiology report. There had not been an abnormality prior to the surgery, and those types of things take years to develop so how had it been there after a forty minute surgery?

Doing what she always did, she turned on the computer to pull up his records. She planned to torture herself over and over, hoping that each time she read it, she might find something new or something obvious which would exonerate her.

Elizabeth waited until the screen came to life. She entered her user name and password. The main screen came up for her electronic medical records. She hit the search bar and entered Frank's name and birthdate, which she had memorized by now. After waiting the customary thirty seconds it took to load, she was shocked when an initial message came up saying,

*You are entering the chart of a deceased patient. Are you sure you want to proceed?*

ELIZABETH PAUSED FOR A SECOND. She had never received this message before. But she wanted to check again, so she leaned forward and hit, *Yes.* Within a second or so, another message appeared across her main screen.

*Access Denied. You do not have the proper permissions to enter this chart. Please see your administrator.*

SHE FELT HER STOMACH CLENCH. Although it wasn't a healthy behavior, she had reviewed this chart numerous times. This was the first time in six months she had been denied access. Her first question was *Why?* It was her patient.

Elizabeth picked up the phone and jabbed the extension for the IT Helpdesk. After being on hold for several minutes, she explained her situation.

"This was my patient and I need to review these records," Elizabeth argued. "I'm being asked to go before a committee to discuss this patient." Elizabeth waited for several seconds for an answer. She listened to the IT consultant tapping on keys.

"I'm sorry," the Helpdesk advisor said. "I'm having difficulty getting this chart to load. It's been restricted for some reason, but I can't see why or who put the restriction in place."

Elizabeth continued to listen to a rapid tapping of keys. After what seemed like hours, she heard him say, "All I could do was send a new password request. It's possible that not all passwords were restricted so pick a new password and try again. I don't have anything else to offer if that doesn't work. You'd have to go to your administrator."

"Thank you, I appreciate it," Elizabeth said as she hung up the phone. She quickly revived her screen and reset her passwords as advised. Once she was into the electronic medical record, she went to Frank's chart and was thrilled when the notes appeared before her. She printed out all she could of the chart in case the computer crashed again. She ran over to the printer, grabbed the papers and stuffed them into her bag.

Knowing pissant Pruitt was after her, she accessed Connie Arturo's chart, printed it out and collected that as well. Just to be certain, she printed whatever she could from Mr. Byron's chart and added it to her bulging purse. She finished printing and read the records on the screen when her access was cut off again. Feeling a surge of panic, and not sure why she would when she should have had complete access to these charts for years, she quickly turned off the computer and picked up her bag. She made her way to the doorway. Looking to the left, she saw Dr. Pruitt exit the elevator and turn toward the medical records room. With eyes wide open, she held her breath as another physician waylaid the good doctor down the hall. When he was occupied, she exited the medical records department and turned right. She scurried to the next cross hall and turned, then turned again as soon as another hall presented itself. Using a circuitous route, she circled the entire floor and finally found her way to a back exit without encountering Dr. Pruitt. She made her way to the car, started the engine and left the hospital property.

# CHAPTER 10

Jake pulled up to the curb in his new, blue Ford Crown Victoria. "Here we go," he said as he looked at the house and property and turned off the engine. The front yard was small, but the lawn was excessively neat and the garden boasted a statue of The Madonna perfectly tucked within a blue grotto. A ring of dark pink impatiens surrounded the ground before the statue. Rose bushes lined the front porch and on the side was a Wisteria tree. There was a hanging plant on the edge of the garden setting off boxwoods under the bow window.

"Looks like a decent home," said Alex. "He must spend a lot of time tending to the grounds. This place is beautiful, looks like a park."

"There's a lot of pride in that property," said Jake.

Alex opened his door. "By the way, how the hell did you get the department to give you a new Crown Vic? The best I could do was a dented Ford Taurus."

Jake laughed. "With so many other cars in use by the department, perps don't look for a Crown Victoria anymore. A new model finally came out and I got the department to dig up the money to maintain my image. Some of my informants are used to a decent level of class. Can't let them down."

Alex rolled his eyes. "I'm your partner, dude. We should both go around in some sense of style."

Jake shrugged his shoulders and popped open the driver's door. "Let's do this."

The pair walked up to the house and knocked on the door. Alex leaned over and rang the doorbell while Jake peered in through the front door window. They waited a few minutes before turning to leave the porch.

"Whatever you're selling, I'm not buying," said a male voice from the side of the house.

The two men turned and saw a middle aged man holding a rake.

Jake stepped forward. "Mr. Arturo? Are you Mr. Arturo?"

"Whoza asking?" The man asked in a very heavy Italian accent.

Jake stepped toward the man. "My name is Detective Jake Wagner, sir. We made an appointment to speak today." Jake held out his badge. When the man didn't respond, Jake pointed to his right and said, "This is Alex Houghton, my partner. We were hoping to meet with you for a few minutes."

Mr. Arturo looked them up and down. "Well, okay," he said as he put the rake down and walked onto the porch. "My name is Pasquale, Pasquale Arturo."

Both Jake and Alex shook the man's hand and offered their business cards. After Pasquale had a few moments to read them, he stepped to the door and unlocked it with a key. He invited both men to come into his home and sit in the living room. They paused for a few seconds, deciding where would be the best place to sit. Jake chose the plastic covered couch while Alex chose to stand near the window. The living room was painted gold with a picture of the Sacred Heart of Jesus hanging on the wall. The windows had both blinds and heavy drapes. There was a St. Anthony statue on a side table with framed photos. Pasquale settled himself in a worn velvet chair and without a smile waited for Jake to begin his questions.

"Mr. Arturo, I'm sorry to have to bother you, but we're looking into the death of your wife, Connie."

"Why?" Pasquale was immediately on guard. "She died in the hospital. What's this all about?"

Jake spoke as gently as possible, "It's about getting information, that's all. Sometimes, we look into circumstances surrounding an unexpected death."

Pasquale's fingers tapped his right leg. "It's that hospital, isn't it? They're afraid I'm gonna go to my lawyer? I should-a do just that."

"Do you mind if we start by reviewing why the surgery was scheduled?"

Pasquale's face clouded over. He leaned over and picked up a framed photo of Connie from the side table. He swallowed hard as he stared at her photo. "My wife, she started having pains in her stomach. She worked hard, Mr. Detective. She was a good wife. She kept the house clean and made a good meal. She went to work every day, too."

"This must be hard for you," Jake said as he looked at Pasquale.

"Every Sunday, she took the time and made perfect homemade gravy."

"Ah, brown gravy," Jake said, trying to connect with the man.

"Whata you mean, brown gravy? She made tomato gravy with macaroni."

Jake heard Alex cough behind him. "I'm sorry, my family always called it spaghetti sauce."

"You, no Italian," Pasquale said waving his hand in disgust at the detective.

"No, I'm sorry, I'm not," Jake apologized. Alex cleared his throat. "Anyway, Mr. Arturo, please tell me about your wife's stomach pains."

Pasquale began again. "She was healthy all her life, then all of a sudden she started having stomach pains. She tried to take a physic but nothing worked, so she went to see that doctor. She's a nice lady."

"Please, continue," Jake coached the man.

"The lady doctor ordered some tests and when they came back, she said that my Connie needed a surgery."

"How did Connie find out about Dr. Brooks?"

Pasquale thought for a moment. "I think she got the name from some of her friends at work."

"Can you tell me where your wife worked?"

"You know, that new building down the street from the hospital."

"I'm sorry, sir. Can you tell me the name?"

Pasquale sighed. "It was MemorHold. She worked there for a few years. They were okay," he said as he shook his hand back and forth. "But they were close so it was easy for Connie to get there and back."

"Did she have any close friends at work?"

"Her boss, Frank," Pasquale said. "She had a girlfriend there too, her name was Deborah."

"Would you know her last name?" Jake asked as he took a small pad from his suit jacket.

"Turner, I think it was Deborah Turner. She came here and gave her condolences, dropped off some food but after the first week, I don't see her no more."

"Does she live nearby?"

"I think she lives a couple blocks away, but I'm not sure." Pasquale shook his head and looked down at his feet.

Jake looked up at Alex and nodded toward the front door. "Mr. Arturo, thank you for your time. We're going to leave now. I'm very sorry for your loss. If we think of anything else, do you mind if we come back?" He stood up and extended his hand. Mr. Arturo shook hands and nodded when Alex said good-bye. When both men were off the porch, Pasquale slowly closed the door as a tear slid down his cheek.

# CHAPTER 11

Elizabeth sat at her desk and tried to review the pile of papers in front of her. The pile consisted of the usual phone messages, prescriptions to be renewed, letters to be signed, and lab to follow up. The staff were gone which was the time of day Elizabeth enjoyed being in the office the most. She was able to get her work done without being interrupted.

Elizabeth settled in her desk chair, went through the lab results and separated them into two piles, one contained normal results and the other needed immediate follow up. She would speak with the patients who needed follow up on their lab tonight and Heather would follow up with the patients who had normal results in the morning.

For the next several hours, Elizabeth spent the necessary time speaking to patients, offering advice for symptom control, calling in prescriptions, and then finally turning to the lab pile. The first results she wanted to see were those of Lucky, aka Mr. John Martin. She rifled through and pulled his results out. She was able to access all she needed on her phone or computer but she insisted on a paper copy so she could write notes and send them to the patient after she called.

Picking up her cell, she called the number listed on his chart. After several rings, she heard someone answer. "Hello?"

"Mr. Martin? Lucky? It's Dr. Brooks. Can you talk?"

After a few seconds, she heard him answer. "Doc? Is that you?"

"Yes, it's me. I have your lab results back. Do you have a few moments to talk with me?"

"Sure, Doc. For you, I have all the time in the world."

"Great, I want to go over your results. Do you want to write this down?"

"No, can we just talk about it and then I'll pick up a copy. I can get the senior bus to drive me over. Gives me something to do."

"Okay, as we suspected, your sugar is higher than it should be. I did a special test which tells me that your sugar, on the average, for the last three months was over 200 on a daily basis. So we need to discuss your diet."

Lucky sighed over the phone. "Doc, food is the only thing I look forward to these days."

"I'm sorry, Lucky, but after looking at your sugar and your cholesterol, you're going to have to find a new place to find joy."

"Well, that's a bummer," Lucky said. "What about my prostate?"

"That blood test is higher than it should be too," Elizabeth said. "I'd like you to see a urologist just to make sure everything is benign. I think you should make an appointment and I'll write everything down for you. My staff can help you make an appointment with the urologist."

"That's nice of you, Doc."

"However we can help, Lucky. Also, I'd like you to bring that new glucometer into the office so I can see what you're doing. We need to get your sugar under control."

"What about my memory, Doc?"

Elizabeth paused for a few moments. "Lucky, I want to get your sugar controlled first. You may feel a lot better and notice you can focus better. To be honest, you haven't shown me enough symptoms for me to believe you have problems with your memory and there's not a blood test to check for that. Let's work on one or two problems at a time."

"Okay, you're the boss."

"Thank you, Lucky. Please make an appointment and we'll work together on a treatment plan. You can try some exercise and diet control for the first three months. If we don't see any improvements, then we'll talk about your medications."

"Sounds okay to me, Doc, but giving up food is gonna be pretty hard."

Elizabeth laughed. "You don't have to give it up completely, but you have to watch your sugar and carbs. You can eat plenty of vegetables and lean protein."

"Yuck."

"Lucky, you have to try it before you complain. Please make an appointment to come in and discuss all this with me."

"I will, and thanks for calling me. You're the only human voice I've heard today."

"You're very welcome," Elizabeth said as she hung up the phone. She felt sorry for Lucky. He was probably a very lonely man. She decided to talk to a social worker in the hospital and see if there were any programs for seniors or veterans that she could recommend to him.

Elizabeth spent the next forty-five minutes following up the rest of the lab results and then cleared off her desk so she could leave for the day.

# CHAPTER 12

"So, what do you think?" Alex asked as they got back into the car.

"The poor guy is grieving," Jake said as he clicked his seatbelt. "I don't think he's involved in her death." He started the car, eased away from the curb and into the roadway. "I think you have an interesting angle we need to explore."

"What's that?" Alex asked as he popped a mint into his mouth.

"The affair. I'm wondering if Frank and Connie had something going on. I don't think Pasquale had a clue if that were the case, but there may have been something more than boss and employee. Do we have any more info on them or the place they worked?"

"I've got some basic stuff at the station. I'll look through it as soon as we get back. Mostly financial stuff from the original complaint, but I'll find more about this company in general. There's definitely a stronger connection then what we've got so far."

Jake started to laugh.

"What's so damn funny?" Alex asked.

"See, that's the reason you're the computer expert and I'm the front guy."

"Get bent, you wad," Alex said as he frowned and crossed his arms.

Alex was quiet for several minutes before he spoke again. "So, what's the doctor's part in this?"

"Not sure, what are your thoughts?" Jake smoothly turned a corner as he navigated toward the thruway.

"Let's assume Frank and Connie were knocking knees," Alex said as he studied his fingernails. "Unless they made a suicide pact, and the good doctor actually agreed to carry it out, I still don't get how she's involved."

"That's the mystery, and the reason the good doctor is going to be the key to break this case. We just have to stay attached to her."

Alex looked at his partner. "She's not going to make it easy."

"No, she isn't," Jake repeated.

"I guess it's a good thing you're the front guy." Alex smirked as he watched the mileposts fly by. "I'm sure your overwhelming charm and allure should dazzle her into telling you everything she knows."

Jake smiled as he moved into the left lane and pressed the accelerator.

# CHAPTER 13

Elizabeth left the office and headed toward home. She finished her work and then called the hospital for an update. Mr. Byron had not yet improved which bothered her all the more since he should have been home by now. She was told his vitals were somewhat stable, except his blood pressure continued to drop slowly. He had regained consciousness but was lethargic. There were no complaints of pain, just sheer fatigue and weakness. His meds were on hold as she didn't want his symptoms masked, although he didn't ask for anything. He continued to need oxygen and his blood levels were stable for now.

Elizabeth knew that Pruitt was watching his recovery just as much as she was. He was waiting for anything to strengthen his case of booting her out of the hospital. He wouldn't be happy until she lost her license, but she hadn't done anything wrong and there was nothing he could prove. She knew of incompetent doctors who never had their technique challenged, much less, their license and integrity.

Pulling into the driveway, Elizabeth decided she would order a whole new set of scans and tests to see if she could identify a problem if Mr. Byron didn't improve by the next day.

She pulled into the garage and turned off the car. The area was dark when she opened the driver's door. The garage light had been working fine the night before. She put the headlights on for a moment to orient herself and then turned them off again. It was amazing how a person carried out the same routine for years but was thrown off in the dark. Everything took on a different cast when you couldn't see well.

Elizabeth gathered her purse and some paperwork she had brought home from the office. She stepped out of the car and slowly made her way toward the door, keeping her hip against the side of the car as a guide. When the back of her legs slipped around the front bumper, Elizabeth took a few steps to the right and stopped where she thought the door should be. Shifting her bundles to her left arm, she slowly reached forward for the door knob but then stopped when she heard a noise. Quietly listening for a few seconds, she didn't hear it again and when she thought about it, she was unable to identify what she had heard. Perhaps a whisper, but not quite.

Once again, she reached for the door knob and turned. When the door opened, she stepped through and immediately turned around, locked the door and shot the bolt. It was odd as she wasn't normally as spooked as she currently felt.

Moving about the condo, she put her things down and took off her jacket. Within minutes, the overhead lights were on, the television blaring background noise and Elizabeth moved into the kitchen to start dinner.

Two days before, Elizabeth had made a shrimp and lobster casserole. Shopping in a new market, she spied a seafood counter which boasted the freshest fish in the region. Upon examination, she had to agree it looked very enticing so she purchased shrimp, lobster and crab. Adding butter, sherry, mushrooms and just the right amount of parmesan cheese, she prepared the casserole over rice. She ate more than she should have on Sunday, enjoying every morsel and now wanted to finish it before the seafood spoiled.

Placing her paperwork in front of her, she plated the rest of the casserole on a glass dish, poured a glass of white wine for ambience and sat at the table. As much as she enjoyed her dinner, she was frustrated at the work she had brought home. Elizabeth had printed out a number of articles dealing with memory loss and prevention in the early stages.

The teaching in medical school was that there were potentially over a hundred different forms of cognitive impairment being researched. For the most part, there were some common causes, but there were also some aberrant causes which had nothing to do with diseases such as Alzheimer's. Mild memory loss may be a normal part of the aging brain and have nothing to do with cognitive disease. If Lucky wanted to pursue that course, she would have to sit down with him and dive much deeper into a neurological history.

Yawning, she put her paperwork aside and brought the dishes to the sink. Once all was washed, the wine bottle corked and placed in the refrigerator, she turned off the lights, checked the doors to ensure they were locked and headed to bed.

Dressed in her favorite nightshirt, Elizabeth settled into bed. To avoid thinking about things over and over, she played soft jazz on her phone, using a sleep timer, in order to help her fall asleep.

Somewhere during the night, she became restless, her body tossed and turned as she moaned. Her eyes flicked back and forth beneath her closed lids.

*THE TUNNEL WAS long and dark. She knew she was in a tunnel and there seemed to be a light in the distance but she didn't know where she was. She wasn't alone, someone was with her. She couldn't see them as much as feel their presence. Beside her, around her, she couldn't figure it out. There was no sense of panic, but she was nervous. "Hello?" She called out as she reached out to her side, her hand touching a cool, damp and slimy wall. She heard a voice.*

*"He's bleeding. You'd better hurry."*

*Elizabeth could hear the words but she didn't see a face. She didn't see much at all as if she were in the middle of a cloud. There was dark haze surrounding her, filling her vision, but the presence lingered. She recognized the voice.*

*"Who's bleeding?"*

*"He's slowly bleeding to death. Save him."*

*Her breathing shallowed. "Frank?" She couldn't grip the image but was sure the presence was Frank Burdette. He had been the first patient to die.*

*"Don't let it happen again. Save him. Save yourself."*

*Elizabeth froze where she stood, the haze around her growing thicker. She realized she was dreaming but couldn't quite grasp the meaning. Now the sense of panic was climbing.*

*"Save him, Elizabeth, while there's still time."*

Elizabeth jumped up and sat on the side of the bed, her heart pounded and sweat dripped down her face. It was early morning, 4 a.m. to be exact, and Elizabeth knew the surgical staff were already beginning to report to the hospital for early procedures. Despite not getting enough sleep, she quickly dressed and rushed out of her home toward the hospital.

She parked in the physician lot and trotted into the hospital, toward the surgical ICU. She burst through the sliding doors and ran to the nursing station.

"I'm so happy to see you here," Elizabeth said as she ran into Caitlyn working at the nurse's desk.

Caitlyn turned and looked at Elizabeth. Caitlyn took note of the wrinkled clothes and wild hair. Grabbing her friend by the arm, she steered her out of the ICU and into the alcove in the hallway. Her voice hushed, she turned toward Elizabeth and blocked her from sight of passing clinicians.

"What the hell is going on?" Caitlyn whispered in a pressured voice as she looked around behind her. "You look terrible."

"Mr. Byron? How's he doing?"

"What?" Caitlyn asked turning back to her.

Elizabeth grabbed Caitlyn by her shoulders. "My patient, Mr. Byron, how's he doing?"

Caitlyn stared wide-eyed at Elizabeth before she spoke. "I just got in, so I haven't examined him yet."

"What about report? Did you get report?"

"Yes, I did."

"What was on report? How is he?"

When Caitlyn didn't respond right away, Elizabeth's stomach clenched. "Oh no, he's dead, isn't he? Did he die overnight?" Starting to panic, Elizabeth raised her voice. "How is he?"

"Stop," Caitlyn said. "You're getting hysterical. He's alive."

Elizabeth sighed deeply. "Caitlyn, please tell me what was on report."

"Okay, I will, but then you better tell me what the hell is going on. I'm starting to get overly concerned about you."

"As opposed to everyone else's gossip," Elizabeth said with a shrug. She continued to stare at her friend as she waited for a response. "Well?"

"Your patient is reportedly the same. His blood pressure is still low and we don't know why. We don't see any blood and he hasn't received any meds which would cause it. We have no idea what's wrong."

"He's bleeding," Elizabeth said. "He's slowly bleeding. That's why you don't see the normal signs."

"How could you know that?" Caitlyn asked as she crossed her arms in front of her.

Elizabeth sighed deeply. "Please don't make me go into it. Let me examine him and order some tests."

Caitlyn grabbed her arm. "Oh no, absolutely not. You are not going into that unit looking like that. If pissant Pruitt walks in, there'll be no coming back. You look absolutely manic at the moment."

Elizabeth was momentarily speechless. She stared at her friend, hurt in her eyes.

Caitlyn softened her grasp. "Listen, please go home, take a shower, go back to bed, drink a pot of decaf coffee." She looked at her watch. "You have to be in your office in a couple hours anyway, don't you? I promise I'll examine him. If there are any issues, I'll order whatever tests you want, even though they're not going to like it in Utilization."

Elizabeth swallowed hard. "I don't care about Utilization. I'm concerned about my patient, not their bottom line or quality data.

Caitlyn, promise me you'll order the tests. Not just if there are issues. I want testing if he hasn't improved. I'll leave for now but only if you promise to put the orders in."

Caitlyn stared at her momentarily. "What do you want me to do?"

"I want Dr. Dillon. Get a consult by Dr. Joe Dillon and I want you to do whatever he orders. He'll need to look at some scans with contrast. Mr. Byron still has good kidney function, right?"

"I believe so," Caitlyn said. "The lab hasn't revealed anything wrong with his kidney function."

"Get a blood count today," Elizabeth said. "He's going to be anemic and he's bleeding somewhere and we have to stop it today. If his kidneys are good, he'll be able to tolerate the contrast. Dillon will know how to fix it."

"We don't normally call in vascular surgeons to deal with complications from abdominal surgery."

"Just do it," Elizabeth said a bit too sharply. "Otherwise, I'm going in there and ordering it in person."

Caitlyn threw her hands up. "Okay, I'll take it as a verbal order, but after this is over, you're going to tell me what's going on. For now, just go home. Get out of here before someone sees you."

"And you'll call me later, with results?"

"Of course, because if nothing's there, I'll want to warn you they'll be out for your head."

"Tell them to get in line," Elizabeth said as she walked around her friend and toward the locker room to get to her car.

## CHAPTER 14

Elizabeth went home, as Caitlyn had asked, and looked into the mirror. As upset as she had been with her friend, she wanted to reach out and hug her when she saw her reflection. Caitlyn, the great nurse that she was, had protected her once again from administrative and judgmental colleagues. They would have been very concerned had they seen how disheveled she was, and if Elizabeth had started ranting about her dream as the motivation for the tests, she would have been placed on leave immediately.

She hopped into the shower, turned the water temperature as hot as she could stand it and washed away the feelings of failure and disgust. After awhile, she was convinced she was as crazy as she felt. Pushed for time, she quickly dressed, dried her hair and left for the office.

Elizabeth was met with a waiting room full of patients and Ruth with a handful of messages. "Your first couple of patients are already in their exam rooms. Here are the important messages, I'll give you the rest after you get started."

Elizabeth rifled through quickly. "Are there any from the hospital?"

Ruth shook her head. "I haven't heard from the hospital yet. But there are plenty of patients who need appointments, have pain or are pending consults that were called in to you. I don't want to promise anyone anything until you look at your schedule and let me know what to do."

"Fair enough," Elizabeth said as she turned and headed toward her private office. She dumped the messages on her desk and placed her purse in the bottom drawer. Opening her computer, she pulled up her schedule and quickly scanned the day's appointments. She flipped through the messages again, walked to the front desk to give Ruth direction and asked which exam room she should start in. Before Ruth could answer, Heather walked by, grabbed her away from Ruth and started to give her report on the first patient waiting to be seen.

Elizabeth pulled the paper chart from the door, scanned it briefly before going into the exam room and pulling up the full digital chart on the office computer. She spent time speaking with the patient, doing her exam, charting her documentation and answering all of the quality questions before she moved on to the next patient.

She followed this routine over and over until the majority of the patients were taken care of. Elizabeth wanted to make sure there was no one left in the waiting room. As she walked toward the front desk, Ruth ran to her, eyes wide and shaking her head.

"What's wrong? Did you hear from the hospital?" Elizabeth's stomach clenched at the possibility of bad news from Caitlyn.

"No, I haven't heard anything from the hospital today, which is very strange."

"Then what's upsetting you?"

"There's someone who asked to see you, but it's not a patient and it doesn't look good."

"What do you mean? Do we need to call the police?"

Ruth swallowed and shook her head again.

"No, I don't think so."

Just then, the door to the waiting room opened. Elizabeth and Ruth looked up to see a male walk into the hall. He was dressed in a tight fitting black T-shirt under a vest with a gold badge hanging from a chain in front of the vest. "Excuse me, are you Dr. Elizabeth Brooks?"

"Yes, can I help you?"

The man took some papers out of his pocket and handed them to Elizabeth with a pen. "Can you sign here, please?"

Elizabeth did as she was told. He then handed her another envelope and said, "Thank you. You've been served." Expressionless, he turned and left the office.

Elizabeth's hand shook as she looked down at the envelope. She turned it over and read the return address. The letter was from a high priced attorney's office in downtown, New Wales. Opening the envelope, she read the letter and started crying.

"Are you okay?" Ruth asked, concerned as the other nurses gathered to see what was happening.

Elizabeth shook her head and swallowed hard. "Not really, no I'm not." She turned, went into her office and closed the door.

# CHAPTER 15

"Dr. Brooks? Are you okay?" Heather waited a few minutes and tried knocking again. "I don't want to leave until I know you're okay."

The door knob turned and Elizabeth opened the door. Her eyes were red and she blew her nose. "I'm fine, Heather. Please don't stay here on my account."

Heather reached out and placed her hand on Elizabeth's arm. "I don't know exactly what happened, but I know you're upset. I don't want to leave you like that. I sent everyone out for lunch so you have some privacy."

"Thank you, that's very considerate," Elizabeth said as she swallowed hard.

"You don't need to be here this afternoon. We only have patients scheduled for their pre-admission testing and bloodwork. I can take care of that with my eyes closed. Why don't you go get some rest?"

Elizabeth was quiet for a moment. "That's not a bad idea. I didn't sleep very well last night so that might be the perfect solution."

"Great. I can call you with any questions or better yet, I'll send an email. That way, if you're sleeping you can answer whenever you get up."

"Thanks, but if I get any calls from the hospital, please make sure I get that information right away." Elizabeth leaned forward and gave Heather a quick hug. "I appreciate everything you do for me."

"You've got it," Heather said as she backed out of the room and closed the door. Elizabeth went to her private bathroom and splashed water on her face. She collected some of the messages she didn't get to as well as her bag. Holding her keys, she left the room from her private back door and walked toward her Audi. The parking lot was empty, except for a new Crown Victoria parked right next to her car. Leaning on it, with arms crossed, was the handsomely dressed Detective Jake Wagner.

Elizabeth unlocked her car and put her things in the backseat. She moved around the detective to open the driver's door, but didn't have enough room without acknowledging the man.

"To what do I owe this displeasure?" Elizabeth asked.

"Just stopped by to say, hi," Jake said.

"By parking so close, I can't get in my car? If you weren't a detective, I'd call the police to report someone stalking me. Since you're out here in the parking lot, I assume you're not scheduled for a blood pressure check."

"True, not today. Although, your nurse was quite adamant I get a recheck within a couple of weeks."

"I imagine she did," Elizabeth said as she pointed to her car door and raised an eyebrow at the man. Jake moved aside which barely allowed enough room for Elizabeth to open the door to slide in. She started the car and jumped a second later, when Jake rapped on the window.

"What?" She asked after she slid the window down.

"You look kind of upset. Are you okay?"

Elizabeth swallowed. "Let's just say I've had better days."

"To be honest, I wanted an opportunity to ask you a few more questions."

"Why am I not surprised? Today is not a good day for me," Elizabeth started to close the window.

"How about tomorrow?" Jake called out.

Elizabeth shook her head, put the car in reverse and backed out of the parking space. After checking for traffic, she turned onto the main road and headed home.

# CHAPTER 16

Elizabeth reached her home and froze. She was still trying to digest the fact she was getting sued and what that would mean to her practice, her license, and her reputation. She knew she should be doing something, like calling her malpractice company, but she couldn't do anything at the moment. Between Dr. Pruitt out for her head and now being subpoenaed she was worried. What more could happen? It was critical that Mr. Byron was okay. What about Connie Arturo? Would her husband pursue litigation as well? Suddenly, Elizabeth panicked - she'd lose everything. Where would she go? What would she do if she lost her practice, license, reputation, pride and faced potential financial ruin?

She sat on the couch, tried to deep breathe and clear her head when her cell phone started to buzz. She saw the hospital phone number pop-up and her stomach clenched. She couldn't tolerate any more bad news, but she was too nervous to ignore the call. What if it were Caitlyn?

Elizabeth picked up her cell and answered. "Hello?"

"Dr. Brooks?" A unfamiliar male voice asked.

"Yes, that's me. How can I help you?" Elizabeth's hand shook.

"This is Joe Dillon, vascular surgeon at New Wales."

"Dr. Dillon?" Elizabeth sat up, more alert now.

"Yes, I believe we've met at a couple of staff meetings."

"I remember. Thank you for calling me. I assume you're calling about Mr. Byron?"

"That's correct. I wanted to talk to you about the case."

Elizabeth's head began to spin.

"Did you see him? Is he okay? What do you think?"

"I assume you haven't heard from anyone else, then?"

Elizabeth's heart started to pound. A question like that could only mean bad news.

"No, I'm not in the hospital today and I haven't spoken to anyone. Can you fill me in, please?"

"Of course, I guess the place to start is to tell you I'm impressed with your diagnostic skills but I'm curious how you arrived at your conclusion?"

"I'm sorry, but you've lost me there," Elizabeth said weakly.

"My fault, let me start over. I just finished performing surgery on Mr. Byron," Joe said.

"Surgery?" Elizabeth froze. "Please tell me more."

"Caitlyn O'Rourke called to tell me of your request for a referral and your suspicion that this patient had a slow vascular bleed. I'll admit I was very skeptical when I got the consult, but I went to see your patient in the surgical ICU. So first, I want to apologize for doubting you." Joe Dillon continued on. "At any rate, I agreed with your assessment of lack of post surgical progress and lowered blood pressure, and of course, the obvious place anyone would look is the fresh surgical site. I obtained several scans and was surprised to find the surgical site was in perfect condition."

Joe paused to collect his thoughts.

"But?" Elizabeth encouraged him to continue.

"The scan did reveal an aneurysm in the renal arterial wall, which had apparently started bleeding. I couldn't believe it because I checked the pre-op scans and saw nothing just as I assume you did. I am unable to explain this, but your patient was stable enough to endure a second surgery where we went in and grafted the area as best we could without interrupting the flow to the kidney. It was tricky and if we hadn't gone in as early as we did, I honestly don't think this guy would have made it. We've escalated his status in the ICU so they're keeping a very close eye on him, but I wanted to congratulate you for picking up that anomaly when you did. Quite frankly, I'm thinking it would be better for you to be teaching my residents than me."

Elizabeth was at a loss for words and mumbled. "I'm glad you saved him." She remembered and repeated the words, mumbled by her dead patient, Frank Burdette, in her dream. *Save him, save yourself.* Elizabeth took a deep breath and repeated to Dr. Dillon. "I'm glad you were able to save him before it was too late."

"I have to tell you, neither myself or my residents would have ever thought of checking this, but it paid off, so I just wanted to let you know, you saved this guy's life."

Elizabeth chuckled softly. "No, I believe it was you and your team who saved his life. I simply suggested it with help from a friend who has had some experience in this area."

"Really? Does your friend have any research to share? I'd be very interested in reading any scientific studies or looking over case studies."

"No, I don't think so," Elizabeth stumbled on her lie. "I mean, I'll ask next time I talk to him, but no."

"That's disappointing," Dr. Dillon said. "I get it. A lot of docs don't want to share any of their data before they're fully published, but this research is fascinating. Hey, do you mind if I present this patient at our next vascular board meeting? It's a great teaching case."

"No, of course not," Elizabeth said. "That would be fine. It's your case now, too. Thanks again, thank you so much for letting me know."

"You're welcome. I'll be following and let you know if we have any complications."

"Great, thank you, Joe. I appreciate it," Elizabeth said as she disconnected the call. She sunk to the couch once more, feeling absolutely numb. She knew something wasn't right. Was it her intuition that morphed into a dream? If not, how could she possibly justify that the ghost of her first dead surgical patient, a man she possibly killed, had visited her in a dream and told her to save her current patient?

# CHAPTER 17

Elizabeth was still sitting on the couch when her doorbell rang. She shook her head, got up and went to the door. Peering through the spy hole, she saw her friend Caitlyn standing on the porch.

Elizabeth opened the door, pulled her friend inside and steered her toward the kitchen.

Caitlyn looked around and saw dirty dishes in the sink. On the counter was a clean wine glass and an open bottle of wine. Next to that was a bottle of bourbon. Caitlyn looked at her friend. "What the hell is going on?"

Elizabeth cleared the counter and gestured to one of the stools there. "Do you want coffee?"

Caitlyn checked her watch. "Sure, I know I told you to go home and take a shower, but I didn't expect you to be home in the middle of the day. Elizabeth, I'm concerned."

"Forget that for a minute." Elizabeth walked back and forth pulling coffee beans out of the cabinet and grinding them for the coffee pot. She filled the reservoir with water, made sure the carafe was straight and turned on the pot. She was glad for the busy work as it helped her focus. Turning toward her friend, she said, "I just got a call from Dr.

Joe Dillon."

"Oh, I'm glad he called," Caitlyn said. "So you know your patient had surgery?"

"Yes, he told me about that and some other things, but I want to hear what happened from your perspective."

Caitlyn shrugged. "Isn't it wild? I went back to the unit and examined Mr. Byron. He wasn't any better and if anything, he was weaker so I did what you asked. I consulted the vascular surgeon as a verbal order from you."

"Any problems with that?"

Caitlyn started to laugh. "You should have seen pissant Pruitt. He was fit to be tied and if he had any real power you would be stripped of your license today."

"What did he say?"

"When he found out you consulted a vascular surgeon and ordered a bunch of scans, he was screaming about utilization and wasting resources as well as pointing out you didn't have the decency to be waiting in the unit for results. He kept blathering until he realized no one was listening to him and then he crawled away in silence."

"Great, I'll pay for that," Elizabeth said as she turned to the coffee pot and pulled out the carafe. She had placed mugs, spoons, cream and sugar on the counter and now filled the mugs with the coffee.

"How did you know I was home?"

"I went to the office to tell you about the results and the surgery. Dillon kept talking about you like you had solved the quantum theory and Pruitt just kept getting angrier, especially when it turned out you were right. He was mumbling something about the case not making sense unless you had known about a problem before the fact and were trying to hide it."

Elizabeth slammed her mug down. "He's an ass."

"That he is. Anyway, Heather told me you went home for the rest of the day. She said I should ask you what was going on."

"Oh really? What else did she tell you?" Elizabeth cringed as she realized the gossip was already starting.

"Absolutely nothing," Caitlyn said. "I swear on my father's ulcer, that's true."

"Hmm, I wonder how your father got his ulcer to begin with." Elizabeth picked up her coffee and frowned at her friend.

"Listen, you know you mean the world to Heather and I. We would never talk about you or rat you out if something were going on, but you've got us scared lately. Seriously, sisters to the end." Caitlyn reached out and placed her hand over Elizabeth's forearm.

Elizabeth choked up within seconds, and tears fell over her cheeks. Caitlyn rushed around the counter and hugged her.

"I'm sorry, Sweetie. I didn't mean to upset you. What's wrong? How can I help?"

Elizabeth looked into her coffee and laughed. She shook her head and searched for the right words to start her explanation. "I went home as you suggested. I showered, dressed and went to the office and saw my scheduled appointments. At the end of the morning session, a gentleman with a badge came into the office and proceeded to serve me legal papers. It appears that Frank Burdette's family has decided to sue me for his wrongful death."

"Oh, I'm sorry, honey. That doesn't mean you did anything wrong. Hell, it's an easy way to make money these days." Caitlyn gave her friend a big hug.

Elizabeth hugged her back. "I think I pissed Karma off somehow. Things were great and all of a sudden, patients are having very weird complications, I'm being sued, and Pruitt wants my ass in a sling. Let's not even get into my embarrassment in front of the staff, patients and anyone else who finds out. And, even though I did nothing wrong, and am considered one of the more talented surgeons by some, I could lose my practice or at least have a big financial headache."

"That's a lot of stress to have all at once." Caitlyn said as she looked at her friend.

"Oh, but there's more." Elizabeth paused to take a shaky, deep breath.

"Okay, I'm waiting," Caitlyn said.

"Did Heather tell you that I'm being stalked by a local detective?"

"What?"

"You heard me. I've had a New Wales detective stalking me. He made an appointment about high blood pressure. When I went to the exam room, he questioned me about Frank Burdette. For all I know he's working for the high priced attorney that's suing me. Then, when I left the office today, he was blocking my path to the car. He said he wanted to talk again, but I refused."

"Is he a private detective?"

Elizabeth shook her head. "No, I looked him up on the internet. He's been with the New Wales Police Department for a long time. He's won several awards as a very accomplished detective." As she explained, Elizabeth showed Caitlyn the screen shot of her research on her phone.

"He's apparently quite attractive as well," Caitlyn said with a smile. Looking at Elizabeth's face, Caitlyn became serious and apologized. "I'm sorry, I know this is frightening." Caitlyn took a deep breath and went on. "To be honest, this morning was very strange. You looked absolutely haunted. Are you sure there isn't more to the story? Have you been dreaming again?"

Elizabeth swallowed hard and began crying again. She put her mug on the counter, got off her stool and turned toward the sink. Caitlyn walked over to her side.

"No one knows about your dreams like I do, so tell me what's going on." Caitlyn stood next to her with her arms crossed, waiting for Elizabeth to speak.

Elizabeth finally looked up at her. "You already think I'm nuts. You're gonna think I'm truly gone if I tell you this."

"Listen, I had to listen to you calling out when you crashed on my couch. I know what happens when you're stressed and tired. If you can tell anyone, it's me."

A few minutes of silence went by. Caitlyn grabbed her friend by the shoulders.

"Elizabeth, I can't help you if you don't talk to me. Tell me what's going on."

"Fine, but then I'm pouring the wine," Elizabeth said as she took a second glass from the cabinet. She poured a glass for each of them and gestured toward the counter stool. "Sit."

Caitlyn did as she was told and Elizabeth slid the wine across to her as she sat on her own stool and took a sip with a shaky hand. After a few seconds, Elizabeth spoke.

"I did have a dream last night. I've been having more of them lately. As you well know, the more stressed I am, the more I dream." She took another sip of her wine. "But last night was different. It's not the first time it's happened that way, but it was different."

Caitlyn's eyes widened as she picked up her wine, but she said nothing.

Elizabeth laughed. "I'll tell you what happened. You don't have to believe me, but I expect you'll never repeat this to anyone."

When Caitlyn nodded, Elizabeth began. "Last night was different than my usual pattern of dreams. I normally dream in all senses. I can see, smell, taste, touch and hear in my dreams. I feel heat and cold and my emotions are heightened." She looked into her wine glass for a moment before she continued. "But last night, it was more of a presence than a dream. I didn't dream of him, I felt him. He was all around me. Hell, he could have been me. I don't know."

"He who?" Caitlyn squeaked out.

Elizabeth giggled. "You'll never believe it, but it was Frank Burdette."

"So, you had a dream about Frank Burdette?"

"Maybe," Elizabeth said. "But it actually felt more like a visit from Frank."

"Wow, and what did he say?"

"He told me that Mr. Byron was bleeding and I should hurry to save him as well as myself."

"What the hell does that mean?" Caitlyn asked.

Elizabeth shrugged, finished her wine and then refilled her glass. "I don't know, but that's when I jumped out of bed, raced to the hospital and found you. It's a good thing too, or Mr. Byron and I would both be in trouble tonight."

"Are you sure it's just not more intense because you've had Frank, Connie and now Byron on your mind?"

"No, this really felt different," Elizabeth said shaking her head back and forth. "And whether you call it a strong sense of intuition, mindful dreaming or whatever else you want, it's a good thing I acted on it."

"Except you looked a bit maniacal," Caitlyn murmured as she sipped her wine.

"Who knows? Maybe I'm nuts and losing my mind just like pissant Pruitt wants everyone to believe."

"Have your dreams intensified of late?"

"Of course, especially since Frank died. I'm totally stressed out. I've gotten nothing but scorn from administration, but the rest of the surgical department has been great."

"Why wouldn't they be? Other patients have died with other surgeons. Things happen at times despite doing all we can."

"Not according to Pruitt. I've apparently ruined all his quality data for the first half of the year."

Caitlyn chuckled. "That's his problem. Let's get back to you. Tell me more about your dreaming. I remember how bad you were when you slept on my couch but I had the impression things had improved."

"They did for awhile, but they're worse of late."

"What about your medicine? I know you haven't been taking it. They have some strong meds for people with sleep disorders and PTSD. Maybe you should try it, at least for a little while."

Elizabeth shook her head. "I don't want to, especially if I have office hours or surgery in the morning. I don't want anything that will make me feel fuzzy."

Caitlyn finished her drink. "Elizabeth, let's be serious, maybe you should see someone?"

"Are you suggesting a shrink?" Elizabeth stood up and placed her glass in the sink.

"No, not necessarily. How about a neurologist or neuropsychologist? There are clear medical reasons why some people dream or suffer intense thoughts in their sleep. Maybe, get a MRI. I don't know."

"I'll think about it."

"And if nothing comes of it, then you can go see a psychic."

"Oh boy, here we go."

"Well, I'm never going to say never. Just in case you've found a way to lift the veil, so to speak. I'm sure people have had some very specific experiences with that as well."

"How about we just let it go for now?"

"What I'd like to do is make sure you can somehow relax and get some rest. The schedule is on the light side right now. Why don't you let the other docs cover surgery and you take a little vacation? Go down the shore and see your parents."

"That may not be relaxing," Elizabeth laughed.

"It may be more relaxing than you think," Caitlyn pointed out. "You don't have to sit with them all day. Go to the beach, watch the water, let yourself relax. You're the only person I know who has access to a beach house and never goes to visit. Take a break, then you can come back rejuvenated and refreshed. I'm serious. Sometimes you just have to get away."

Elizabeth considered her suggestion. "I'll see. I want to go in and see Mr. Byron tomorrow. I'll have to make some calls to my malpractice company. Then I'll think about it."

"Promise?"

"I promise," Elizabeth said as she gave her friend a hug.

"Good. I'm going home. As you well know, I started with a very early shift today. I'm about to pass out myself."

Elizabeth walked her friend to the door. "Get home safe and I'll talk to you tomorrow." After a few seconds, she said, "Thanks for being a friend."

"Anytime, Sweetie. Anytime."

# CHAPTER 18

Elizabeth cleaned the kitchen and decided to lie down. She was tired from her dream the night before, the emotion surrounding Mr. Byron's surgery, and the rest of the day.

Elizabeth felt guilty to be napping, but she was exhausted and depleted, physically and emotionally. Despite being late afternoon, she changed into comfortable bed clothing, turned on her fan, closed the blinds and snuggled under the covers. Within minutes, she was sound asleep.

She slept deeply, and then woke around 1:00 a.m. She had slept for six or seven hours and woke up somewhat refreshed, although nowhere near enough to get up for the day. She turned on her side and tried to fall back to sleep, but slowly tortured herself with thoughts of her lost patients, the lawsuit, pissant Pruitt, and Detective Wagner. She was glad that Mr. Byron was stable, at least she hoped he was and not having any more problems. Just the mere thought that a patient had died under her hand took her breath away. After Frank coded in the unit, she hadn't slept well for months. Her anxiety grew on a daily basis and she thought about leaving medicine. However, once the investigation was concluded and his cause of death was certified as an aneurysm, she realized it had nothing to do with the surgery. She was so thankful when she read the coroner's report, she had wept. Several months later, the same thing happened to Connie Arturo. Once again, she sweated it out, checked and rechecked the records. There was nothing on the pre-op testing which would lead someone to believe Connie had a potential vascular problem. Those images had been checked by multiple physicians since then, so they were not read incorrectly. The facts did not make sense. Now with Mr. Byron, she had to wonder if there was something else going on, but she still couldn't justify the pathophysiology.

Elizabeth got up and without turning on the lights, went to the bathroom. She washed her hands, drank some water and then returned to bed and fluffed her pillows. She repositioned herself in bed and tried to clear her mind for sleep. After tossing and turning and noting it was now 3:00 a.m., she finally used her phone app to start playing soft piano music. Setting the timer for 45 minutes, she recited the rosary. She could tell she was drifting off to sleep due to the random thoughts which were entering her mind.

*She was standing in a field. She stared at tall green grass dotted with wild flowers. The day was pleasant and warm. A breeze caused the grass to sway and blow around her. In the distance, she saw several trees. The leaves fluttered with the wind. Within seconds, the sky turned dark. Elizabeth continued to stand there and look up at the sky. She quivered with the electric energy one feels right before a heavy rain. At first, a plump rain drop fell on her face. Then several others fell around her, on her head and arms. She could see the wall of rain advancing toward her. Elizabeth walked toward the trees. She was getting soaked as she walked and hoped the trees would shield her but she paused when she saw a figure under a branch. She drew a little closer and saw a man standing there. He was leaning against the trunk of the tree, his arms crossed over his chest in front of him. His legs were crossed at his ankles. He rested there, watching her. She wasn't able to see his expression. Elizabeth continued to walk as the rain grew heavier and lightening now appeared in the dark sky. Thunder answered in the distance as the wind blew her wet hair and damp clothing around her. The closer she drew to the tree, the more anxious she became. Suddenly, she realized the man beneath the tree was Frank Burdette. Elizabeth stood there in the rain, indecision causing her to freeze. Looking to her side, the thunder and lightening drew closer. Her hair was plastered to her face, her clothes were soaking wet. When she looked back, Frank continued to lean against the tree trunk, staring at her. She couldn't decide what to do. She tried to measure each threat against the other and simply couldn't move. A bright flash of lightning lit the entire sky, blinding her to details around her. The bang of thunder caused her to jump up in bed, heart pounding, struggling to figure out where she was and what was happening.*

ELIZABETH SAT on the side of her bed for several minutes, trying to wake up and reorient herself with her room. She knew from her training in medical school that she was in a hypnogogic state, the transitional period between wakefulness and sleep. She often had hypnogogic jerks as she fell asleep. As she drifted off, a part of her body would suddenly spasm or jerk in response to a thought or image that crossed her mind. Usually, she would dream she was falling when she would startle and wake up. If she was immediately able to clear her mind of the dream long enough to relax and change her thoughts, she would be able to fall back to sleep for a while more.

That's exactly what Elizabeth worked on at that moment. And finally, leaning to her side, Elizabeth fell back and nestled her head on her pillows. Within minutes, she was asleep and stayed that way until early morning.

# CHAPTER 19

The next morning, Elizabeth awoke, but stayed in bed for a few minutes. As usual, she reviewed her thoughts and especially the dreams which stayed within the edge of her thoughts for the first couple of hours in the morning. There had been times when she retained a dream for hours until it was replaced by the busy moments of the day. But the images and places she dreamt of seemed to call out to her as she felt sleepy and got ready for bed the following night. She clearly felt as if she were being called back to a certain place by night, while working in the world during the day. And in her dreams, she was usually "somewhere", getting ready to return home. She was confused as to how she was going to get there, but she realized she wasn't home.

Elizabeth got up, showered and dressed. She grabbed her phone and bag and headed toward the hospital. Parking, she went into the hospital through the locker room and straight to the surgical ICU. She was grateful the OR schedule didn't have an opening for her until the following week. Mr. Byron was now three days post op and she wouldn't have to worry about anyone else for awhile.

Stopping at the nurses's station, Elizabeth observed the monitor signal coming from Mr. Byron's room. She waited until his assigned nurse approached the station.

"Hi, Deidre. How are you?"

"Hi, Dr. Brooks. I'm well. How have you been? Long time, no see."

"Yes, I've been here but it appears we've been on different shifts. I see you're taking care of Mr. Byron?"

"That's right. Very nice man."

"Can you tell me how he's doing today?"

"Oh, sure," Deidre said. "She turned to the computer and pulled up his record. She reviewed all testing and consultation with Elizabeth. "He's doing much better since he had the second surgery. He had a transfusion of packed cells yesterday. Dr. Dillon was very happy with the results of his CBC."

"That's great to hear," Elizabeth smiled.

"His vitals are good, he's alert and oriented and his dressings are dry. So, I think we're finally on our way."

"I'm happy to hear you say that," Elizabeth said. "I'm going to go in and see him."

"He'll probably be ready to transfer to a step down today or tomorrow. Do you want to give the order or should I call Dr. Dillon?"

"Please call Dr. Dillon. Since he did the last surgery, he's in charge. I'll agree with whatever he suggests."

"You've got it, Doc."

Elizabeth picked up her bag and made her way into the ICU cubicle. The patient was lying in the bed, his head turned to the side as he was looking out the window. His wife sat in a chair next to him.

"Hi, Mr. Byron," Elizabeth said as she approached his side. "How are you feeling today?"

He turned to face her. "Hey, Dr. Brooks. How are you?"

"I'm fine, but the question is, how are you?"

"I'm feeling a lot better today. I've got a lot more energy than yesterday. To be honest, I've lost some of the last two days. I don't know if it was the medicine or a poor recovery. What happened?"

Elizabeth smiled as she answered the very delicate question. She turned to him and said, "I'm not completely sure. The surgery you had with me was fine. We removed your gallbladder and were able to sew you up and get you to ICU. You didn't recover as quickly as I expected which is why I asked Dr. Dillon to do a consultation. He discovered you had a weak vessel near your kidney, which was bleeding, so he fixed it and now you're getting stronger."

Mr. Byron blew out a sigh. "Well, I'm sure glad to hear that."

Elizabeth sat next to the bed and placed a hand on his arm. "If you don't mind, I'd like to ask you a question."

"Sure, Doc, go ahead."

"I went over your records very carefully before you went to surgery. I looked at all your medications and supplements. I was a bit concerned because you bled more than you should have during surgery and that didn't involve the kidney problem yet. Are you sure you told me everything you were taking, prescription or otherwise?"

"I'm pretty sure. I mean I'd have to take a look at the records to see if there's something I forgot to tell you about but I'm pretty sure I wrote it all down when I filled out the initial papers."

"Okay, I was trying to figure out why you might have bled more than usual. Do me a favor. If you think of anything you might have left out, please let me know?"

"Definitely, I will. I don't need any more problems, Doc. So, is this it? What's the next step? Am I gonna get out of here soon?"

"I certainly hope so, but Dr. Dillon is going to be in charge of you from this point on. I'm going away for a few days, so he'll write all of your orders and then discharge you when he feels everything is stable."

"Then what do I do?"

"Well, you'll have to see both of us for follow up. I'm going to want to see you in the office next week and he'll have to follow up with some testing of his own."

"As long as I'm out of the hospital, that's cool." He nodded as he listened to her instructions.

"Okay, remember, when he sends you home, you'll call my office and make an appointment to be seen. Okay?"

"You've got it, Doc. Cross my heart." He made an X over his chest as he said the words to Elizabeth.

"Okay, great. I don't expect to have to come back and see you here so I'll see you next week in my office, but if you're still in the hospital on Monday, I'll come back and visit. I'm so glad you're feeling better."

"Me too, you have no idea." He nodded his head to emphasize his words.

Elizabeth squeezed his hand and then left the cubicle. She went to the nurses station and spent a few minutes writing out last minute orders in the computer. Elizabeth then called Joe Dillon. He agreed with her plan to have him discharge Mr. Byron when he felt the kidney graft was stable. At least Elizabeth was confident that Mr. Byron was in the care of a gifted surgeon.

As she left the ICU, she went to medical records to write a final note on Mr. Byron. Using the new passwords she had obtained, she was able to bring up the chart in the electronic medical record and transfer service to the vascular surgeon. She also printed a complete copy of the records for herself.

Once Elizabeth was done with the chart, she tried to call up Frank and Connie's charts but neither would come up for her again. Grateful she had printed everything out on her last visit to medical records and before she received the notice from the attorney's office, she had immediately made additional copies for her office and her home. Her plan was to review the hospital records as well as her own as she was sure they would all be called in for the discovery process.

Taking her copy of Mr. Byron's chart, she logged off of everything and left the hospital. She drove to her office, entered her private door and placed all the records in a safe place. Within minutes, she heard a knock on her door.

"Come in," Elizabeth said.

"Hey, how are you?" Heather asked as she walked into the room. "I wasn't sure you'd be here today. Caitlyn called to tell me you were pretty stressed."

"Very true, but I was able to get some sleep last night," Elizabeth said with a small smile. "Even so, you've both suggested I take some time off and I haven't taken a vacation in six months, so I'm taking you up on your offer."

"Really?" Heather was shocked. "You never listen to us. What's different this time?"

"I think you're both right. I haven't done anything wrong and I have nothing to hide, but the stress is not letting up and I think a couple days off might help me refocus."

"That's great to hear," Heather said as she realized how her words sounded. "I mean, I think it's a great idea. Not that I want to get rid of you or anything."

Elizabeth laughed. "Sure, when the cat's away…."

"Trust me, there's no mice here."

"Will you be able to reschedule my patients? I'll be back to work Monday morning. I'm just taking a long weekend. Also, I signed Mr. Byron's case over to Dr. Joe Dillon so he's taken care of as well."

"Okay, sure. I'll go check the schedule and help Ruth now."

"Thanks, I appreciate it. I have a few calls to make and then I'm going to leave. You have my cell. If anything critical comes up, call or text me and I'll get right back to you."

"You've got it boss," Heather said as she left the room. "Have a great time."

"Will do," Elizabeth said. She spent the next 15 minutes making some very important phone calls, then left the office to go home and pack.

# CHAPTER 20

"Find anything?" Jake asked his partner as he walked into the squad room.

"There's quite a bit of information on MemorHold," Alex said as he slid his chair back and pointed to his computer. "But it's all scrubbed. This is the squeaky-clean version the public is allowed to know about."

"That's great, but we need the other version," Jake said. "How about the dark web? Did you try that yet?"

"Going there, next," Alex said. "Trying to get my game on. What about the good doctor? How did today's visit go?"

"Nowhere," Jake said. "I got there at 4:00 p.m. but Dr. Brooks was not in the office. They had some other guy filling in for her today. Apparently she isn't going to be around for a couple of days."

"Is that coincidental or is something else going on?"

"I don't think it was planned. When I called for an appointment the other day, I was given Friday as a choice. Today is Thursday and suddenly she's not available for several days. Something's changed in the schedule."

"Maybe the schedule was busy and she just took a couple of days off."

"Could very well be, but I wonder what she's doing with those days. I went by her place and waited outside for 30 minutes but she clearly wasn't there. What information do you have on MemorHold?"

Alex shrugged his shoulders. "The clean stuff is that it was formed in 2016. It's a supplement company that claims it has a product which can help preserve memory and prevent dementia. I haven't read any of the studies yet, but they're on my list. It's a multimillion dollar company and apparently somewhat aggressive in terms of their marketing. Both Frank Burdette and Connie Arturo worked there before they died."

"Who owns it?"

"Don't know that yet. It looks like a shell company owned by another shell company, but I was able to find a CEO by the name of ....," Alex rooted through several stacks of paper until he found a card. He picked it up and read, "name of Phil Harry."

Jake started to chuckle.

"What's so funny?" Alex asked, frowning.

"You've heard the old adage?"

"Guess not." Alex shrugged.

"Never trust someone with two first names," Jake said with a laugh. "Get a chance to look him up yet?"

"Just preliminary information. I didn't find a criminal record under that name, but I didn't find anything else either. No up and coming announcements in business magazines, no history of achievements on Wall Street, as a matter of fact I couldn't find a credit card."

"Interesting," Jake said. "What about a driver's license or a social security card?"

"Nothing yet but I just got everything together. I'll need another day, then we can go out there."

"Not yet. Let's not spook anyone," Jake said. "Take another day to do some research. Also, I want to know more about Deborah Turner, Connie's friend."

"I can try to look her up tomorrow," Alex said. "I may have to resort to extraordinary methods."

"I'm sure you'll find her with no problem. Besides, I'm not

comfortable being aggressive while the doc's in the wind. If she's truly taking a break, she should be back by Monday morning. They're not going anywhere if they don't know we're watching."

"If there's anything going on in the first place," Alex said with a scowl.

Jake slapped him on the shoulder. "There's always something going on, buddy. You know that."

# CHAPTER 21

Elizabeth walked to her car with her luggage in tow. After making sure all her patients were covered, she went home and packed for the weekend. She made one last call to Caitlyn and Heather to let them know where she would be.

As she pulled out her dresser drawers, looking for bathing suits, cover ups and shorts, she realized she hadn't been swimming for at least two years.

Elizabeth had grown up on the Jersey Shore in a beach town named Misty Point. The population was approximately 1000 in the winter and swelled to 25,000 in the summer. It was a great beach town, mostly owned by a woman named Rose Stanford. She was a kind woman who lived in a beautiful Grand Victorian named Misty Manor, which sat on the North Cape of Misty Point. Elizabeth was sure she had been in the same high school as Rose's granddaughter, Megan, but she honestly couldn't remember a lot about her except that Megan graduated a few years after her in school. One of Elizabeth's favorite places was the lighthouse the Stanford family had built in the early 1900's, which was still active to this day.

The feelings of nostalgia surprised Elizabeth as she anticipated seeing her home town, Misty Manor, the boardwalk, the beach and the ocean again. When she was in college and medical school, she would love going home when she was overwhelmed and enjoyed the healing effects of the sea. The vast ocean and beautiful weather always helped her put her concerns in perspective and after a few days of rest and relaxation, she was ready to return to her life.

She took the ramp and guided her car onto the Garden State Parkway. It was only Thursday and she was hoping it was too early in the season to hit traffic. Once summer hit, traveling south on the Parkway usually meant patches of bumper to bumper traffic. That was okay as it would give her time to clear her mind and focus. She always did her best thinking in the middle of the night, when all else around her was quiet, unless, of course, she fell asleep and started to dream. Driving during the day, in a quiet car, had the same effect. There were times when she wished she could just keep going without choosing a specific destination.

Her parents, C.J. and Parker Brooks, had lived in Misty Point since they married and vowed never to leave. Over the last 35 years, their small beach house had grown in size and value, but that had nothing to do with their love of the shore. Elizabeth's room remained the same as it was in college and was open anytime Elizabeth wanted to return.

C.J. and Parker both enjoyed spending a good part of the New Jersey winter as snow-birds in Florida. Parker was a retired physician who spent years taking care of patients near the beach. He was also trained in Sports Medicine which came in handy with all the walks and races held on the boardwalk. They had three children of which Elizabeth was the youngest. Elizabeth had two older brothers, but she hadn't seen them in several years. They were both married with children of their own. As Elizabeth pulled into town, she wistfully thought of how nice it would be to have the entire family together again. She planned to speak to her parents about setting up a reunion soon.

Elizabeth drove down Main Street and smiled at the sight of the ocean on her left. She opened her car window and enjoyed the scent of salty air, combined with suntan lotion and grilled food. It was early in the season and the temperature was perfect. Within minutes, she was pulling into the driveway of her family home.

As Elizabeth pulled her luggage from the car, her parents walked out of their Cape Cod and down the stairs to meet her. Her mom reached her first and wrapped her in a tight hug. "Oh Lizzie, it's so good to see you."

"Hi, Mom," Elizabeth said as she hugged her back.

"This certainly is a pleasant surprise," her Dad said as he hugged her about the shoulders. At his feet a dog pranced around and whined.

"Thanks, Dad," Elizabeth said as she leaned over to pick up her bag. "Whose dog is that?"

"Oh, this here is Goldy," Parker said as he scratched the ears of a beautiful Golden Labrador Retriever.

"Is he yours?"

"Well, we sort of adopted him."

"You got a dog? And you didn't tell me?"

"It was a surprise to us," C.J. explained. "The animal shelter had a problem and they asked residents to temporarily adopt the pets until they reopened the shelter."

"But when it was time to bring her back, we thought she might like to stay a while more," Parker shrugged.

Elizabeth dropped to the ground and hugged Goldy as the dog spent several minutes licking Elizabeth's face.

"I love her. She's so gentle."

"Golden Retrievers are a favorite breed for patients with disabilities. They're frequently trained to help blind patients or those with autism who need a therapy dog. A good police dog, too."

"She's beautiful," Elizabeth said as she continued to nuzzle the dog.

"How was your trip?" Parker asked as he picked up her bag.

"Not too bad. I didn't hit any traffic."

"That's great. You have to leave at just the right time."

"Well, I guess I did," Elizabeth said with a smile.

Her mother caught up to her and squeezed her arm. "Lizzie, as much as we want to believe you're here because you totally missed us, we thought you sounded a bit stressed on the phone."

The trio walked toward the house and up the stairs as Goldy followed behind.

"Yes, work has been a bit crazy lately, so I thought a weekend at the shore, with my parents, would be the best way to relax."

"That's so nice to hear. We're happy you'll be with us for the weekend. I freshened up your room for you. Why don't you get yourself settled? We'll have dinner around 5:00 p.m. Is that okay with you?"

"It sounds wonderful, Mom," Elizabeth said as she started toward the stairs. Both of her parents watched her walk up the flight toward her room. When they heard the door close, C.J. turned toward her husband.

"I don't know, Parker. I have a bad feeling about this."

"Oh, you and your feelings. The poor girl needs some rest."

"She hasn't been sleeping again. I can see it in her face. There's something big going on."

"Well, if there is, can you give her five minutes to at least unpack before you get on her back?"

"Hush up, Parker, or I'll get on your back." C.J. shot him a pointed look. "I'm worried about her. She had such a hard time going to all those doctors. I'd feel bad if it started all over again."

C.J. didn't wait for an answer before heading to the kitchen to begin dinner. Goldy stood in the foyer and whined as she tried to decide what to do.

C.J. prepared a nice green salad and took fresh burgers from the fridge. When Parker peeked in to see what was happening, she handed him a plate of raw burgers and fresh vegetables as well as the spatula he would need for the grill. He whistled for Goldy and the two went outside to cook. C.J. concentrated on setting the table and opened a bottle of wine to let it breathe.

Just to be sure it was a good choice, C.J. poured a small glass of wine while she was waiting for Elizabeth to come down for dinner. Twenty minutes later, Parker and Goldy came back into the house with a platter full of grilled burgers and vegetables.

"Is Lizzie here?"

"She hasn't come down yet," C.J. said as she poured another ounce into her glass. "Maybe you should go up and check on her."

Parker scowled, but they both turned their head when they heard footsteps on the stairs. Goldy wagged her tail.

"Here she is," Parker said as he embraced his daughter when she neared the table. "It's so good to have you here."

"Thanks, Dad. It's nice to be here."

"I hope you're hungry. Dinner is ready if you'd like to sit at the table." C.J. ushered everyone to the table and they chose their usual seats. Goldy took up a position under the table so she'd have the best view of any hands holding out a small bit of food.

C.J. placed all the platters of food on the table, picked up the wine bottle and paused over Elizabeth's glass. "Would you like some wine? It's a nice bottle of Moscato."

Elizabeth nodded. "Sure, thanks."

C.J. poured for Elizabeth as well as Parker and herself and then sat at the table. She passed the platter of cheeseburgers and grilled vegetables. Then she passed the salad. "Your father's cholesterol has been climbing so we're eating less meat and concentrating more on vegetables."

Parker rolled his eyes and quickly frowned at Elizabeth, who smiled in return. Although she wanted to ask her Dad if he was okay, she hesitated to bring it up at the dinner table.

"So, how are you?" Parker asked as he cut his hamburger in half and took a generous portion of salad. "Is everything okay?"

C.J. kept her eyes on her plate as she waited for the answer.

"As I said, things are a bit stressful at the office, so I'm taking a small break. I've had a couple of difficult cases recently and I want to clear my mind so I can focus on the details."

"That sounds like a good idea, and we're happy to see you back home," Parker said as he bit into his burger. "Do you have any specific plans for tomorrow?"

"No, haven't even thought about it," Elizabeth shook her head. "Knowing me and how early I get up, I'll probably go walk along the beach for a couple miles in the morning."

"It's supposed to be a beautiful day," C.J. said.

"Maybe I'll walk to the lighthouse. I haven't been there for awhile. How is Mrs. Stanford?"

C.J. put her fork down. "Oh, honey, we haven't had a chance to talk to you about her, but she passed away over a year ago."

"Really? I'm sorry to hear that. She was a nice lady. So, what's going to happen to Misty Manor?"

"You'll never believe who's back in town. Megan came back to care for Rose at the end. She's such a sweet girl. Anyway, after Rose passed, I think the whole town turned out for her funeral. Makes sense since she owned over half the town anyway, but Rose was such a kind and generous woman."

"Then a week after she was buried, Rose's no good son showed up thinking he had a get rich quick scheme by selling Misty Manor."

"Oh no," Elizabeth said. "Misty Manor has been there for a hundred years. So, what happened?"

"Well, I'm happy to say, as far as I've heard, Megan inherited her grandmother's estate as well as her philanthropy positions. Her father gave up and left. Thank goodness."

"Wow, that's a lot of change," Elizabeth said. "I haven't seen Megan since high school. We weren't very close back then but I hope she does well."

"So far, so good. The Stanford Foundation is the main support for the animal shelter. Last year, the veterinarian, Dr. Arnie Stokes, was shot and they had to foster all the pets until they got a new veterinarian which as you've heard is how we've come to love Goldy. She's such a good girl. Megan did a great job keeping the shelter open so I believe she'll continue doing good things."

Elizabeth chuckled. "I haven't been to the ocean yet, but I already feel better about my problems."

The small group was quiet as they ate their food and slipped small pieces to Goldy. After a few moments, Parker cleared his throat and said, "You know we're always here if you want to talk about anything. We're not totally demented, yet."

"Thanks, Dad," Elizabeth said as she reached out and squeezed her father's wrist. She grabbed her mom's as well to make sure she knew how much she loved and appreciated both of them. "Maybe, I'll tell you about it tomorrow."

"I hope you'll be having dinner with us tomorrow night," C.J. said. "John Donovan is coming over and I know he'd love to see you."

"I haven't seen John in awhile," Elizabeth said.

"He's been busy at the funeral parlor," Parker said. "Ever since his wife died, he's immersed himself in his work. We're trying to get him back into the world of the living."

Elizabeth laughed despite her mood. "Yes, dealing with the dead can be rather disconcerting at times."

C.J. picked up her wine glass, side-eyed her husband and decided to stop at the liquor store first thing in the morning.

# CHAPTER 22

Elizabeth woke the next morning to a perfect day. Through the opened window she heard seagulls calling out to each other as waves pounded toward the shore. The house was not directly near the beach, but when the ambient noise was quieted, it was close enough to hear the ocean. Once the day began, the sounds would represent trains, lawn mowers, and garbage trucks. Then, as the day wore on, the sounds would be replaced by laughter, music, beer bottles being pulled from an icy cooler, and yard parties, until the noise died down once again. The humdrum of daily life at the shore was so very different from being in the city.

Elizabeth relished the smell of the shore as well. Instead of going into the hospital with the smell of antiseptic, cleansers and disease, Elizabeth couldn't wait to jog to the boardwalk for the smell of salt air, suntan lotion, and eventually grilled burgers with fries and cotton candy.

Goldy had slept on the bed with Elizabeth and now spent the morning trailing after her to the bathroom, the closet and downstairs to the kitchen. Elizabeth wanted to run before she began eating or drinking so she stretched and planned to head out immediately.

Goldy was waiting by the door and whined as she watched Elizabeth stretch.

"What's wrong, girl?"

More whining as the dog flicked her eyes up to the leash hanging by the door frame.

"I get it, you want a walk?"

The second Elizabeth said the word, the dog sprang to her feet, wagged her tail and looked hopeful. After a few seconds, Elizabeth grabbed the leash.

"Oh, what the hell. You have a leash, so I assume they take you out." Attaching the leash to her collar, the two headed out. "I hope you like to run a little."

The pair walked up the street until they reached the boardwalk. Elizabeth took in the gorgeous view of the sandy beach and ocean. The waves were bold this morning, with a pleasant cool breeze and the warm sun to fill the day. It was too early to worry about a beach pass, so they walked to the packed sand near the water's edge. Turning north, Elizabeth looked down at the dog and said, "Let's go."

They jogged at a decent pace and after a while Elizabeth realized she could drop the leash. Goldy followed her with an occasional side trip to the water, but the pair stayed together for a mile or so.

Elizabeth stopped to rest and gazed at the lighthouse in the distance. It hunkered there, keeping watch over the distance as if it were a guardian of life and the sea, and in reality, it was. Time flew by rapidly and Elizabeth realized she had been in this very spot hundreds of times in the last thirty years. During that time, the lighthouse, the coast, the ocean had remained rather solid, unspoiled and a great bastion of focus. Problems seemed small and timeless when in this spot.

They turned around and ran south until they reached their starting point. Goldy darted back and forth, playing with a few waves while Elizabeth walked to loosen her muscles.

"C'mon, girl. We'd better get back to the house and quite frankly, I'm looking forward to a great cup of coffee."

With Elizabeth holding the leash, the two of them left the beach and headed toward the house.

"There you are," Parker said as he turned from the stove. "I'm making bacon. Have you eaten yet?"

"No, not even coffee. We went out for a run this morning. I wasn't sure if Goldy was trained, but she was great."

"I'm sure she loved it. I wish I could take her out but my arthritis has been acting up a bit. You should come by more often, if not for us, for Goldy's sake," Parker said as he flipped several pieces of bacon in the frying pan.

"After a beautiful run this morning, I'm sorry I haven't been back more often." Elizabeth unclipped Goldy's leash and hung it near the doorframe. She walked into the kitchen to continue talking with her father. "To be honest, Caitlyn pushed me to come down here. Things are so stressful in the office and hospital."

"I got that feeling when you arrived. You looked tired. I know I'm retired from practice, but I've had a lot of experience, good and bad, while I was seeing patients. If there's anything you ever want to talk about, I may have an interesting insight."

"I know, it's just so hard to discuss."

C.J. was almost to the kitchen and stopped short when she heard them talking. If Elizabeth needed some space to open up, she didn't want to break the moment so she backed up and went into her bedroom.

"Honestly, why don't you run it by me?" Parker turned off the frying pan as he placed the final slice of bacon on paper towel over a paper plate to drain the grease.

He turned toward his daughter and said, "What do you think?"

Elizabeth immediately burst out in tears. "Oh, Dad, I've lost two patients."

Parker hugged her tightly. "Okay, it's okay. Let's work this out. Let's go out on the porch and tell me what's going on."

As the two went outside to sit and talk, C.J. wandered into the kitchen where she poured several mugs of coffee and stole one of the bacon slices off the plate. Her heart burst inside to see one of her children hurting, but she didn't have the resources to help her with this problem. Parker was the right person to talk to. She put the coffee on a tray and decided to wait a few more minutes before she brought it out to the porch. It was a gorgeous day and it was perfect weather to have coffee outside. She pulled a few muffins from a dessert box and placed them on the tray along with some locally made jelly. Picking up the tray, C.J. walked out to the porch and quietly placed their coffee and muffins in front of them as Elizabeth explained her situation to her father.

"The two patients died in post-op and the strange thing is the anomaly they died from had nothing to do with the surgery either time. I reviewed the pre-op labs and X-rays over and over. When the mortality review was done, everyone agreed the abnormalities were not present on the pre-op films so it's not like I missed an obvious problem."

"And the radiologist read the film the same way?"

"Yes, there was nothing there to cause us to change or cancel the procedure."

Parker reached out and patted his daughter's knee. "You know, doctors are not perfect, things do happen."

Elizabeth sniffed and laughed at the same time. She used the back of her hand to wipe snot away from her nose. C.J. immediately leaned forward with a napkin.

"That may be true, Dad, but unfortunately, the Chief of Surgery wants to use those two deaths to throw me out of the hospital."

"Who? Pruitt?"

"That's pissant Pruitt to you, Dad."

They both stopped to chuckle.

"He always was a horse's ass," Parker said as he leaned forward to pick up his coffee. "Don't forget, when someone's agenda is self-serving, they'll use anything to further their cause. Stand strong, concentrate on facts and you'll be fine."

"I certainly hope so, because I feel him gunning for me."

"So now that we all agree you're not responsible for any of these deaths, the question is have you figured out what's going on?"

"I have no idea," Elizabeth said as she picked up her coffee and took a sip. "I'm at a loss."

"The first thing I would recommend is to pull all the charts, all the medical information and comb through it to find commonality."

Elizabeth thought for a moment. "You know, now that you mention it, there was one weird thing."

"What are you thinking about?" Parker asked as he continued to sip his coffee.

"I have to be honest. I've been eating myself alive, day after day, rereading the chart, looking for something I missed and I can't find anything. But a strange thing happened. The other day, I went to read the chart for the ten thousandth time and suddenly access to the chart was denied."

"Oh?" Parker asked as he raised an eyebrow.

"Yeah, something's not right. I called IT and they gave me a temporary password so I printed out as much of the chart as I could."

"That's an excellent idea," Parker said. "Who knows? Maybe it's an IT issue because they flagged the chart for review. Why don't you send me the printed copies and let me go through them? As an outside observer, maybe I'll identify something that's not obvious."

"That would be great, Dad. It would be nice to have someone with a medical background, other than me, read through the charts."

"I would relish the opportunity, Pumpkin, especially if it would help you out."

Elizabeth smiled as she took her father's hand. "At minimum, it helps me think I'm not alone in this. You have no idea how important that is, knowing you'll have my back, no matter what the outcome is."

Parker smiled. "Family is family and don't ever forget that. I know what my family is capable of. I trust in that, not in someone's opinion."

Elizabeth leaned forward and hugged her dad and then hugged her mom. "You have no idea how important it is to hear you say that. Coming here was definitely the right decision."

"Damn straight," C.J. said as she lifted her coffee mug to her lips.

# CHAPTER 23

Elizabeth spent the day doing some of the things she enjoyed most while growing up in Misty Point. She donned a bathing suit for the first time in years. She then grabbed an old beach bag from her closet, stuffed it with beach towels, suntan lotion, and a good beach-read. Stopping in the kitchen, she added water bottles and several snacks to her bag. As she left the house, she tossed a casual, "Goodbye, Mom. I'm headed to the beach." She laughed as the comment brought back a host of memories from high school.

Walking two blocks to the beach, Elizabeth stopped when she reached the boardwalk and looked around. Her mom had a house beach tag that she used to get onto the sand so she didn't need to go to the beach hut.

Elizabeth walked toward her usual spot and enjoyed looking at all the sand castles along the way. Every year, the town held a contest and there were no holds barred. The talent and skill were amazing as the various artists created their masterpiece. Small prizes were given out as well as photos posted on the town website for the season.

Walking past several volleyball games, she found her space and spread out her blanket. Elizabeth enjoyed being closer to the ocean to enjoy the breeze and small splashes of water as the tide came in.

She took time to evenly apply her suntan lotion, while watching swimmers slowly ease into the waves. She enjoyed the breeze on her face, the briny smell of the ocean, and the warmth of the sun. After 10-15 minutes of quiet observation and soul searching, she pulled her beach-read from her bag and opened to the first page. It had been awhile since she took time to read a book and she enjoyed being able to escape from her thoughts and worries.

Several hours later, Elizabeth came to consciousness. In the distance, she heard the drone of an airplane, children laughing and music. She was on her side and it took several seconds for her to realize she was still on the beach, on her towel.

With the breeze moving her hair about her head, she kept her eyes closed and listened to the waves rush to shore. She had been reading and felt sleepy, and now realized she must have fallen asleep. It had been a long time since she had had the luxury of waking up on the beach after a long nap. She was at peace, for the moment, and didn't want to move.

Elizabeth realized she hadn't slept well since her first patient, Frank, had died. Her insomnia worsened and then the dreams restarted. Enjoying her small respite, she was thankful for her long, but more importantly, dreamless nap. If sleeping on the beach was the only way she could have restful, peaceful sleep, she vowed to make a habit of it.

Walking home, Elizabeth stopped at her favorite fudge store. Using her credit card, she bought four pounds of fudge, all mixed flavors. She'd leave one pound with her parents, bring one home, another to the office and one just for Caitlyn. Elizabeth was glad she'd followed Caitlyn's suggestion to take a few days off. She felt better already. Pissant Pruitt and the attorney's office seemed far away right now, although her stomach clenched as her thoughts briefly touched on her problems. She had a little more time before she had to go back north and was determined to enjoy it.

Elizabeth grabbed her beach things and her fudge and walked back to the house. Entering the laundry room door, she immediately smelled a delicious aroma and noticed their dinner was cooking on the stove.

"Elizabeth? Is that you?" C.J. walked into the laundry room. She held a dish towel in her hands. "I was worried."

"Thanks, Mom." Elizabeth said. "I can't believe it, but I fell asleep on the beach."

"Really?" C.J. took her daughter's beach towel and put it in the laundry basket for the next wash.

"Yes, and quite honestly, it was the most peaceful few hours of sleep I've had in a long time."

C.J. smiled as she looked at her daughter, although her eyes welled up with tears. "I'm so sorry things have been hard for you lately. You went through so much when you were young. I swear if I could go back and punch that drunken driver in the head, I would."

Elizabeth hugged her mom. "It's not your fault. Things happen, sometimes."

"But if I had run faster, if I could have pushed you out of the way of the car..,"

"Mom, please stop. There was nothing you could do."

C.J. shook her head. "You wouldn't have had to go through all the surgery, the neurologists, the mockery."

Elizabeth wrapped her arms around her mom and whispered in her ear. "Please, let's not do this now. One day we'll talk it all out. There's a lot of pain, but let's leave it buried for today. I just need to relax."

C.J. swallowed hard and nodded. "Okay, when you're ready."

"Just know that I don't blame you and I never will," Elizabeth said. "Let it go. Stop blaming yourself." Elizabeth let her mom go and grabbed a clean towel. "I'm going to run upstairs and take a shower."

"Okay, but remember John Donovan will probably be here when you come down to dinner."

"I'll make sure I'm presentable." Elizabeth chuckled as a nose pushed in the laundry room door. "Goldy, how are you, honey?" The dog ran to Elizabeth's side and nuzzled her neck when Elizabeth dropped to a knee in order to hug her better.

C.J. shook her head. "That dog is in love with you."

"She's a beautiful dog," Elizabeth said as she stroked her coat. "I've thought about getting a dog, but it wouldn't be fair considering the amount of time I'm away from my place. I might be able to sneak her in the office, but I definitely couldn't do it in the hospital."

"Then you'd better come visit more often to see her. It will get you away from your practice and help you to relax."

"I may just do that," Elizabeth said as she gave the dog one last scratch. "C'mon, girl. Let's go upstairs."

# CHAPTER 24

"We just got a hit on her credit card," Alex said as he tapped on his keyboard. "She's at the Jersey Shore."

Jake spun around on his beaten chair in the squad room. "I knew she wouldn't go far. She's not the type to run. I bet she just had to blow off some steam. There's a lot going on and things seem to be warming up."

Alex continued to search the web. "Apparently, she's got family down there. Looks like she's back in her hometown. Oh, this is interesting. Her dad is a retired physician. Her parents remain married."

"See? She's going home for the weekend. A good daughter checking on her parents."

Alex shook his head as he continued to surf the web. "I'm looking for more information on the CEO, Phil Harry, and MemorHold. Are we still waiting for Monday? Then why the hell am I here on a Saturday? I should be on the beach."

"Stop whining," Jake said as he stood up and pulled on his weekend suit jacket.

"Go to hell," Alex said. "Now what?"

"C'mon, let's buzz by MemorHold. I want to scope out the building and neighborhood while no one's around. We'll wait to meet Mr.

Harry until Elizabeth returns. I still think she's going to be the key to this mystery."

"Okay, we case the place, then I'm out until Monday morning. You can work eighty days in a row because you have no life, but I have things to do."

# CHAPTER 25

Elizabeth turned off the shower spray and stepped onto the bath rug. Goldy rushed forward and licked the warm water off her leg. Grabbing a towel, Elizabeth wrapped her hair and then used another Turkish towel to wrap around her body. She leaned forward and patted Goldy on the head.

"You are a sweet girl."

The dog rubbed her head against Elizabeth's towel and wagged her tail.

Twenty minutes later, Elizabeth and Goldy descended the stairs into the living room. The table was set and Elizabeth saw her father and John Donovan in the living room having a pre-dinner libation.

"Elizabeth, how are you?" John asked as he rose from the couch and walked over to offer a bear hug.

"Hello, John. How are you?"

"I'm doing fairly well. I was sharing my thoughts with your father," John said as he stepped back.

Parker Brooks had practiced medicine in Misty Point for many years. He had a lot of summer residents but also took care of year-round residents. There weren't many funeral parlors in Misty Point, so after years of having patients die naturally, and numerous death certificates to fill out, he had become fast friends with John Donovan, the son and director of Donovan and Son Funeral Parlor.

Parker took care of John's father when he developed acute leukemia years back. Parker sent him to a cancer center for treatment but when the time came he was also the one who discussed his goals and thoughts and wishes for the end of his life. Parker made sure he was comfortable and helped the rest of the family through their grief. For that, John has always been grateful, but the men found a common bond in good food and great literature which kept them together.

"Elizabeth, would you care for a glass of wine before dinner?" Parker waited by the kitchen counter for her answer.

"No, I think I'll have some water for now. I fell asleep on the beach and I feel a little dry."

"Water's a good idea. Hydrate. You'll feel much better." Parker tossed a cold bottle of water to his daughter.

Looking back and forth at the men, Elizabeth said, "You two look like you're up to no good, as usual."

"Nah, we were just sharing some of our favorite stories," John said.

"Oh yeah? Like what?" Elizabeth drank from her water bottle as Goldy circled her feet.

John looked at Parker and laughed. "I feel bad, but do you remember when you were a little girl? I used to come to the house to get the death certificates signed. That was way before they were on the electronic system."

Elizabeth narrowed her eyes. "Vaguely, why?"

"I didn't realize it at the time, but I always drove over here in the hearse to get your father's signature."

"Was the recently deceased inside?" Elizabeth asked, eyes wide open.

All three turned when they heard C.J. mutter, "Oh Lord," and pour herself a glass of wine.

John shuffled his feet and looked down at the floor.

"Really? You had the body inside the hearse?"

"In all fairness, that only happened once. I was in a rush to get the permit filed with the town and your father was partly to blame because he kept me in the waiting room for an hour."

"Well, I didn't know you had Mr. Weathers in the hearse."

John let out a hearty laugh. "If you'd come out to ask, I would have told you. Your patients took pains to walk on the other side of your driveway that day."

"Yes, and as I recall, you were here so long, one of my neighbors called to see if we had a tragedy in the family. I'm sure it didn't do much for my patients confidence either."

John picked up his drink and continued to laugh as Elizabeth stared thoughtfully at the wall. Goldy, sensing her angst, pressed her nose against Elizabeth's leg.

C.J. walked to the edge of the living room and cleared her throat. Looking at Parker and John, she said, "Gentlemen, and I use the word loosely, why don't we come back to the land of the living and sit down for dinner?"

"If it tastes as good as it smells, this will be a fine dinner," John said. "You always make a great meal, C.J."

Elizabeth and Parker smiled, walked over to the table and took their customary seats. Goldy settled at Elizabeth's feet, under the table.

"John, you are such a charmer," C.J. said."And don't think I don't know it. You'd say the same thing if I made peanut butter and jelly sandwiches."

"True, you got me there," John said with a laugh. "But you are a great cook. If I wasn't friends with Parker, I'd compliment you a lot more."

Parker reached out and squeezed his wife's hand. "Unfortunately for you, John, I am here." Looking up at his wife, he said. "She is a great cook."

"Lord, it's warm enough," C.J. said. "All this hot air is killing me. Okay, watch out. Our first dish is soup, Lobster Bisque."

"That sounds great, Mom," Elizabeth said.

"Next we'll have a Caesar salad, with fresh bread and butter, then pan seared scallops with fresh mozzarella and sliced prosciutto, and for dessert, we have coconut sorbet."

"Well, I'm impressed," Elizabeth said.

"I think you'll enjoy it," C.J. said. "Ever since your father retired, I've been spending more time learning to cook."

"Why since he retired?" Elizabeth asked.

"Well, after you left for college, when your father's practice was still active, he'd never make it home for dinner. I'd make a new recipe but had no one to try it out."

"That's not true," Parker said. "You'd bring the dishes to the office."

"Yes and quite a few to the neighbors," C.J. laughed. "But food tastes much better when it's freshly served, so let's eat."

The group sat and enjoyed the meal, making small talk throughout.

John turned to Elizabeth toward the end of the meal, "How are things in New Wales?"

Elizabeth nodded. "It's busy, I'll say that."

"Life seems much busier north of the bridge," John said referring to the Driscoll Bridge, a toll bridge on the Garden State Parkway."

Parker cleared his throat. "As a matter of fact, Elizabeth was just telling me about a case conference she was involved in."

Elizabeth shot her father a warning glance but Parker subtly shook his head.

"Really? Anything interesting?"

"It seems there's been a slight trend toward vessel anomaly after surgery or in some of the posts they've been doing. I was just wondering if you've seen anything like that lately?"

"Parker," C.J. admonished.

"Well, sorry honey, it's just that John sees a lot of pathology as an embalmer. We're just inquiring if he's seen any unusual patterns."

"Wonderful, I think I'll be doing the dishes now." Elizabeth felt bad when her mom left the table. She would have helped her, but wanted to hear John's answer.

"It's interesting you say that, Parker. You know we have a few different techniques to embalm depending on how the patient died. I mean we usually use the right common carotid artery and the right internal jugular vein, especially as we don't have to worry about arteriosclerosis there as much. I know you're aware that hardening of the arteries always raises the risk of pressure causing leakage and tearing in arterial walls. Sometimes, we use Single-point injection but lately, we've been forced to use Multi-point injection most of the time to prevent blowing the features."

C.J. walked in on the last several words, gasped, immediately turned and went back into the kitchen. She stopped for a second and called the dog. "Goldy, come eat." All three heads turned and watched her go with the dog following behind.

John then leaned forward and kept his head to a whisper. "As you know, we have to use Multi-point injection whenever we have a body that needs low pressure injection. You know the six points. Right leg, left leg, right arm, left arm, the trunk and then the head separately. Anyway, we're getting a lot of older patients who all seem to have some sort of vessel problem so everything has to be done using Six points."

John turned to Elizabeth. "What was this conference about? Did they identify anything specific?"

Elizabeth swallowed as she stalled for a few seconds. "Actually, it involved two cases of surgical patients who died of vascular abnormality after the surgery, but the area involved was no where near the surgical field."

"That's exactly what I keep hearing. It's as if the people's vessels have become mushy in general. That's very strange and maybe it's more of a trend than we think. Maybe you should call the State and have them collect some data to see if they could track these abnormalities. You may be onto something big."

C.J. cleared her throat. "Can I please come in now?" She was carrying a tray with a coffee pot, mugs, cream and sugar.

"Of course, C.J.," Parker said as he shot up and took the heavy tray from her.

"Thank you," C.J. said. "I have to go back to the kitchen to get the sorbet."

Parker put the coffee tray on the table and turned back to help C.J. when she appeared in the doorway with four glasses of chilled Coconut Sorbet. She placed one at each person's place sitting.

Elizabeth had started pouring coffee for all. Knowing how her parents preferred their coffee, she automatically spooned in cream and sugar. She asked John his preference and then after pouring his, she sat down.

"Thank you, Elizabeth," John said as he turned to C.J. "And I want to tell you how delicious this meal has been. I'm not just being nice, this was a great meal. I'm sorry about the table talk, but we're done now."

"I appreciate that," C.J. said. "I suppose I should be used to medical shop talk by now, but the older I get the more it bothers me."

"Mom, it's gonna be hard to have two doctors in the family who never discuss the industry. There are so many changes in treatment as well as process and policy, it's the best way to keep everyone up to date."

"I know, I know," C.J. sighed. "If you have to, do what you must. I just hope we get to do some fun stuff, too."

Parker crossed his heart. "We're done for tonight, I promise." As C.J. spoke with John, Parker turned to Elizabeth and mouthed, "We'll talk more later."

# CHAPTER 26

After they finished coffee and dessert, Elizabeth helped her mom clear the table, wash the dishes and close the kitchen for the night. John Donovan said goodnight and left the Brooks family standing at the door. The night was warm with a gentle breeze.

"Hey, what say we take an evening walk up to the boardwalk like old times?" Parker suggested as he looked at the women.

"Sounds good," Elizabeth said as she looked at her mom. "Can we bring Goldy?"

"I don't see why not," C.J. said as she reached for the leash.

"I've got some money in case we want to get a drink or a cone." Parker fumbled with change.

"Great, let's go." Elizabeth bent forward and hooked Goldy to the leash.

The four of them set out towards the boardwalk. They walked on the sidewalk to avoid any problems with drunk drivers.

"I haven't done this for a long time," Elizabeth said, her hair blowing in the breeze. "I forgot how gorgeous the full moon looks hanging over the ocean."

"Truth be told, we don't go as often as we should," C.J. said. "When you live somewhere full time you stop appreciating the reasons other people flock there to begin with."

"I don't see how you couldn't go out on a night like this," Elizabeth said. The small group made their way onto the boardwalk and walked south. Goldy was well behaved and didn't jump at other beach lovers out for a walk. After ten minutes or so, they found an empty bench and sat down to rest. While there, they heard a thunderous boom and realized they were lucky enough to catch a fireworks display for the weekend.

Elizabeth reached down and covered Goldy's ears, but she didn't seem to mind too much. She did push her head toward Elizabeth's leg and didn't move as Elizabeth held her. Fascinated by the beautiful splashes of color in the sky, the group didn't move until the grand finale was over, with hundreds of different colors exploding at once. "That was beautiful. They've come a long way with fireworks, the colors and patterns were glorious."

"Yes, they sure have," C.J. laughed. "When your father and I were dating, it seemed like there were a few basic colors."

"I think they were still using TNT back then, Dear," Parker chided. C.J. smacked him in the arm.

Elizabeth suddenly yawned. "Oh wow. I can't believe I'm tired after I slept on the beach."

"Yes, but you've not slept well for several months now," Parker said as he looked at his daughter.

"You know me too well," Elizabeth said.

"That's why we want to make sure you're feeling okay," C.J. said. "You're tired because the adrenaline is wearing off as you let yourself relax. We know what happens when you're stressed."

Elizabeth nodded. "And I am very stressed. I'm still stressed, but somehow, coming back home, and to the shore, helps put things in perspective. Caitlyn was pushing for me to take a few days off and I'm glad she made me leave the hospital. She talked to Heather who made arrangements for me to be out of the office." Elizabeth was quiet for a few moments. "They were right."

"Well, I think the information John talked about was very important, Elizabeth," Parker said as he dodged his wife's pointed look. "I won't go over it all, but it will be important for you to look into what we discussed when you go back north."

Elizabeth nodded without commenting. Goldy pulled on the leash and the group started walking again.

"What about that ice cream?" C.J. asked, making a face at Parker.

"I'm in. I haven't had a good ice cream cone since last summer. Lizzie, you want ice cream?"

Elizabeth felt a wave of melancholy as her dad called her by his favorite nickname. "You know, I think I would like that."

Fifteen minutes later, the group silently walked home while licking their ice cream cones and wiping their mouths with tiny white paper napkins. They arrived at the house and everyone, including Goldy, slowly walked up the stairs onto the porch.

"I'd love to sit outside for awhile, but I'm kind of beat so I'm going to go straight upstairs," Elizabeth said.

"We understand," C.J. said. "Sleep as much as you can. How about an old-fashioned breakfast tomorrow? We can have scrambled eggs, bacon and pancakes? I have some fresh strawberries as well, with whipped cream."

"Sounds great, Mom." Elizabeth bent forward and gave her mom and dad both a kiss on the cheek. "I'll see you in the morning."

"Good night, Lizzie."

Parker and C.J. watched Elizabeth go into the house. Goldy followed her inside. They both took a seat on the porch swing and were quiet for a few moments.

"What do you think?" C.J. asked, weariness and fatigue accentuating her question.

"Just what we said," Parker replied. "She's very stressed right now. She's at a critical point in her practice and her profession. I'm glad she got away and came down here to relax. I'm not sure we answered any questions for her, but we may have given her a starting point."

"I wish she had a loving husband who could take care of her at night. He could help her set limits, eat properly and get some sleep."

Parker was silent for a few moments. "We both know she's married to her profession, like most doctors are. Plus, she's afraid to have a relationship. I know what she's thinking. Why bother dating someone just to have them find out about her ability and leave."

"Ability or disability?" C.J. shot back, anger in her voice. "It must be very hard on her, not having someone close to rely on, especially when she's troubled."

"I know. I know," Parker said as he took his wife's hand in his. "But someday, she'll find him. Mr. Right is out there and he'll support her."

Choking up, C.J. squeezed his hand. "I sure as hell hope so."

# CHAPTER 27

Elizabeth undressed and spent time in the bathroom getting ready for bed. She couldn't believe she was so tired but her mom was right. For the first time in months, she was allowing herself to relax. She didn't feel as vulnerable staying with her parents and having to fight every emotion, every thought, while flogging herself for things out of her control.

Approaching the bed, she pulled down the light covers. She opened the window for the breeze, knowing the air conditioning wasn't on. The night was cooling off and most times, Elizabeth enjoyed the fresh air near the ocean. When it quieted, she could hear the crash of the ocean waves which helped lull her to sleep.

When Elizabeth sat on the bed, Goldy looked up at her with big questioning eyes. Elizabeth smiled, the dog jumped up on the bed and waited for her to stretch out. Goldy then turned a few circles and plopped down at her side, stretching her body to match Elizabeth's form in the bed.

With the breeze blowing the curtains into the room and the fan moving the cool air around, Elizabeth turned off the light and let herself drift off to sleep, her hand resting on Goldy's side.

Two hours went by and the pair naturally turned a bit while they slept. Goldy woke first and stared at Lizzie who began to moan in her sleep. Sensing something was wrong, Goldy put her head on her paws and whined.

*She was walking on a path. The path was wide and there were trees on both sides. Elizabeth knew it was daytime, but she couldn't see much except the dirt path before her and the trees to the side. Elizabeth continued to slowly walk forward. She couldn't describe her emotion. It wasn't stark fear, but more of a weariness as she didn't know where she was or why she was there. Up ahead, she saw Frank walk out from behind a group of trees. He was waiting for her, and he was smiling. He nodded as she approached.*

*"You finally found the right path," Frank said.*

*"What path?" Lizzie asked, looking straight at him. He looked healthy, happy and younger than when she remembered meeting him.*

*"The right path, just keep going. Not gonna say it'll be easy, but you can't go around it, can't go over it and you can't go under it. You gotta go through it, but it'll be great when you reach the other side."*

*Lizzie felt herself getting nervous. "Frank, what are you talking about? Am I gonna die? Is that what you mean? Is that what it's like when someone dies?"*

*"Didn't say that, I just said you finally found the right path and you should keep going no matter what happens." He turned around, and walked away while whistling a popular fifties tune.*

*"Frank, come talk to me," Lizzie said as she got frustrated. She looked down as she felt something wet drip off her hand. She was afraid she would see blood, but when she dropped her gaze, she saw Goldy licking her fingers. The dog kept nosing her hand and licking her fingers.*

Elizabeth woke with a start. She remembered her vivid dream despite feeling slightly confused, but when she looked at her side, Goldy was there licking her hand. When the dog noticed her looking, she immediately raised up on her paws and licked her face. Elizabeth hugged the dog to her and took a couple of deep breaths as she let the dream fade away.

After a nightmare, she normally wouldn't be able to fall asleep for hours as she rehashed the meaning over and over, but Goldy distracted her by putting her head on Elizabeth's shoulder and nuzzling her on the cheek. Elizabeth felt herself slowly relax and within fifteen minutes was sound asleep once again until she awoke the next morning.

Daylight shone through the window and Elizabeth could sense the time was later than usual. She rolled over and saw it was 9:00 a.m. Elizabeth hadn't slept that late in years. Her first impulse was to jump up, but then she realized she didn't have to be out of bed, especially when she saw Goldy's sad face. Elizabeth relaxed back down onto the pillow and hugged Goldy to her side as she softly spoke to her.

# CHAPTER 28

Twenty minutes later, Elizabeth walked down the stairs and spied her parents in the dining room. Her mother was pinching the ends off the crispy pieces of bacon her father had cooked. C.J. would pop a small piece in her mouth and take a sip of coffee.

Elizabeth walked to the table and sat with Goldy at her feet. "I can't believe I slept so late, but it felt great." As she said it, the memory of her dream hit Elizabeth. Maybe Frank was referring to her getting more sleep. She did feel better than she had felt in months. The dreams were so frustrating when she didn't know if they were meant to be literal or not.

C.J. passed the bowl with the scrambled eggs and then the platter with bacon. "Here you go."

"Thanks, Mom. It's been such a long while since I took time off from my practice, I'd forgotten how other people live."

"Then you better make it a point to do it more often," C.J. said. "Toward the end of your father's practice, I made him take a week off every quarter." She held her hand up, palm facing outward. "Oh, he didn't want to do it and fought me tooth and nail, but eventually he found it was better to pace himself then have a stroke and be of no good to anyone."

Elizabeth looked at her father who frowned and shrugged at her at the same time.

"What plans do you have for today, Pumpkin?" Parker asked. "Anything special you'd like to do?"

"I can't say that I have anything special in mind. It's probably important just to take a good nap, maybe finish my book." After a few seconds, Elizabeth looked up and said, "Maybe we can take a ride to Lighthouse Drive and watch the ocean from up high."

"Sure, that sounds like a great idea," Parker said. Clearing his throat, he asked, "Are you planning on going back tomorrow?"

Elizabeth nodded slightly. "Yeah, I've got to work this out. Something's amiss, and I feel more strongly than ever it's not me, so I have to figure it out."

"I can't keep quiet anymore," C.J. said as she shook her head. She reached out and covered Elizabeth's hand. "Tell us, are you having dreams again?"

Elizabeth looked at her mom. "Are you sure you really want to know that? Whether I am or I'm not, it's just going to upset you either way."

C.J. looked down at the table and swallowed.

Elizabeth reached out and patted her mother's hand. "Why don't we leave it at I need to rest. Right now, I'm at a low point, physically, emotionally and spiritually. If I relax, sleep and keep eating at this pace, I'll be twenty pounds heavier by Monday, but I'll probably feel a lot stronger."

"Okay, let's make plans for today," Parker broke in. "When do you want to leave for Lighthouse Road?"

Elizabeth shrugged.

"Great. C.J., let's clear the table and get the dishes done. Lizzie, you bring Goldy outside and make sure she does all her business. She hasn't left your side since you got here. We'll all touch base in forty-five minutes or so and get ready to take a little drive." Parker turned to Lizzie. "In the meantime, if you think of anything else you'd like to do before you head north tomorrow, then let us know as soon as possible so we can work it all together."

"Thanks, Dad," Elizabeth said with a smile.

The trio spent the rest of the day enjoying themselves. In the evening, Elizabeth felt the anxiety begin to creep back in as she settled in bed, but Goldy, still at her side, nuzzled her shoulder. Elizabeth turned slightly and stroked her head.

"Hey, were you raised as a therapy dog? I'm wondering because you seem awfully good at what you're doing this weekend."

Goldy sighed loudly and rested her head on Elizabeth's arm. Within minutes, they were both sound asleep.

Eleven o'clock the next morning, Elizabeth placed her bag in the back seat of her car along with two large bags of food her mother had packed for her.

"I wish you could stay all summer, Pumpkin," Parker said as he gave his daughter a big hug.

"I do, too," Elizabeth whispered near her father's ear. "I had a nice weekend, some extra sleep, great food and fun in the sun. Plus, I had my own therapy dog."

"Yeah, I'm a little worried about how she's going to react when you leave," Parker confessed. "Is there any way you can come back next weekend and straighten her out?"

Elizabeth smiled. "I don't want to make any promises. I have no idea what I'm gonna find when I go back to work, but I promise you I'll be back sometime this summer."

"Better make it sooner rather than later," Parker said as he stepped back.

C.J. moved forward and hugged her daughter tightly. "If anything, this weekend made me realize how much we miss you. Please come back, soon."

"I will, Mom," Elizabeth said as she gave her a big hug. Elizabeth turned toward the car and right into the sad eyes of Goldy. Elizabeth dropped to her knees and hugged the dog around the neck. "Oh, girl, I'm going to miss you a lot." Goldy licked her face several times and whined. When Elizabeth tried to get into the driver's seat, Goldy strained her leash trying to jump in the car. Parker had to exert a good bit of effort to hold her back.

"You'd better just rip off the band-aid and go. This is not going to be pretty," he said as he pulled the dog back once again. Elizabeth closed the car door as Goldy began barking and whining.

With a knot in her stomach, she put the car in gear and slowly pulled away from the house. Several minutes later, she turned toward the Garden State Parkway with tears coursing down her cheeks.

# CHAPTER 29

Dawn broke early Monday morning and Elizabeth reluctantly slipped out of bed and into the shower. She dressed and arrived at the hospital twenty minutes later.

Parking in her usual spot, she went into the hospital through the locker room, put on her white coat, and headed to the surgical ICU.

She walked to cubicle number five and felt her stomach drop when she saw the bed was empty. She walked into the cubicle just to make sure the patient wasn't out for a test, but confirmed that there was no current patient.

Elizabeth realized she hadn't had the energy to call over the weekend to check on Mr. Byron's status. She didn't check in with the hospital or with Caitlyn. Once she heard he was stable from Dr. Dillon, she transferred him and wrote him off her worry list, but now that she wanted to check on him, he was gone.

Elizabeth hurried out of the cubicle to find Caitlyn. She checked at the front desk only to find out Caitlyn wasn't scheduled to work.

Stumbling over her words, she backed out of the ICU, and over to the cafeteria to get a cup of coffee. Elizabeth wanted to get to the back corner of the physician's section and make a private call to Caitlyn.

Pouring the steaming beverage into her cup, a group of surgical residents walked into the café and began loading plates with fruit, bagels and pastries. Surgical prep often began by 5:00 a.m. with early scheduled procedures and the staff waited to eat until after their first several cases were done. Elizabeth couldn't help overhearing their conversation.

"I can't believe the size of that tumor this morning. I don't know how anyone can walk around with something like that without pain."

"I'm sure there was discomfort, but some people are scared of surgery. They'll hold off until they don't have a choice."

"Amazing."

"Did you hear there was another death in surgical ICU this weekend?"

"Yeah, I can't believe it. The State Department of Health is gonna be in here soon."

Hot coffee scalded Elizabeth's arm as the liquid spilled from the cup. She quickly placed the cup on the counter so the residents wouldn't see how hard her hands were shaking. She gripped the counter so the dizziness wouldn't cause her to fall as her heart rate shot up and her chest constricted.

"From what I heard the patient was fine and then suddenly crashed. They were there immediately but he didn't make it."

"Yeah, well I attended that code and it was nasty. They were trying everything. It was weird, the patient was fine one minute and then suddenly bled out."

Elizabeth couldn't tell if the resident voices faded because they walked away or if she were passing out. She continued to grip the counter, frozen in time.

"Are you okay?"

Elizabeth turned toward the male voice at her side.

"Are you okay? You look mighty pale."

Elizabeth let out a weak laugh as she spied one of her colleagues next to her. "Oh, I was getting coffee and got a little dizzy."

"Did you have anything to eat yet? Maybe your blood sugar is dropping."

"No, I haven't eaten yet."

"Here, let me help you get some coffee. It looks like you've scalded yourself. Let's get a plate and go sit in the doctor's lounge."

Dr. Bruce Covington helped Elizabeth pour another cup of coffee and fill a plate with eggs, bacon and buttered toast. He put the plates and coffee on a tray and carried it back to a table. Guiding Elizabeth to a chair he waited until she sat. "Have some protein. I'm sure you know as well as I do, it will stabilize your sugar better than a carb."

Elizabeth smiled and prayed she didn't begin sobbing in front of this man. "Thank you. I appreciate your help."

"What about that wrist?"

Her gaze followed his to the red piece of skin that she now realized was burning like hell.

"I had a hot cup of coffee in my hand and I got dizzy. The coffee sloshed out and burned my wrist."

Bruce shook his head. "Isn't it amazing? Some days the coffee is nuclear and the other days cold. Anyway, after you eat, you'd better go over to central supply and get some cream on that before it begins to blister up."

She looked down and nodded. "I'll definitely do that. It's starting to burn."

"Eat first," Bruce said as he pushed her plate closer to her. "You have any cases scheduled this morning?"

Elizabeth shook her head as she chewed. "No, I was just coming in to do rounds before I go to the office."

"Good, then you have plenty of time to eat and get fixed up before you see patients."

As Elizabeth ate, she realized she was hungry which might have made her less able to hear bad news. She needed to hear what happened as soon as possible. She needed to get to Caitlyn.

"Yes," Elizabeth said. "I'm feeling better already. Thanks for being so kind."

"I've been a surgeon for thirty years. Our profession has one of the highest burnout rates ever and it's getting worse. Always happy to provide a hand." He laughed at himself. "Please excuse the pun."

Dr. Bruce Covington was a respected surgeon in the hospital.

Always pleasant and calm, he had served as past Chief of Staff. His wife of twenty five years and children were very proud.

"Thank you for that. Apparently, it's needed at all levels. I do appreciate your concern. Please let me know if there's anything I can do for you." Elizabeth smiled her appreciation.

"Will do, now back to work and you go get some cream."

Elizabeth sighed as she watched the surgeon clean his tray and walk out. He was right, she needed to get some burn cream, calm down and talk to Caitlyn. Getting hysterical wouldn't change anything now for the poor patient.

# CHAPTER 30

Using a burn gauze, Elizabeth smeared a generous amount of cream on her wrist. She then securely covered the wound with more gauze and paper tape. Slipping her white jacket on, she found the sleeve covered most of the bandage but the wound still burned.

Taking a deep breath she pulled out her phone and dialed Caitlyn. After several rings, her voicemail came on encouraging her to leave a detailed message and have a pleasant day. "Call me as soon as you get this. I came home last night so I'd like to get caught up with things. I don't know where you're assigned today, but I'm going over to my office. Call me."

Elizabeth left the hospital and drove to her office. She parked and went in through the back door. She wasn't surprised when she spied a large pile of charts, lab and messages on her desk. The office had been covered by another doc but they mostly handled emergencies, not the routine stuff. Elizabeth liked it better that way as she often made complex decisions and treatment plans with patients. Having someone else come in and change things midstream could be more disruptive than helpful.

The door to her office opened and a harried Heather walked in with two more charts. "Oh, I didn't realize you were back. I was going to organize your desk pile, but I haven't had time. We took care of some of the messages but there's still things you have to follow up on."

Elizabeth walked around her desk and sat down. "Thanks, Heather. I just arrived so I haven't looked at a thing, yet. I stopped by the hospital earlier in the day. Have you gotten any messages from there?"

Elizabeth waited and was surprised when Heather shook her head. "No, nothing much from there. You don't have any cases scheduled until next week and there's no one in post-op right now."

"What about Mr. Byron?" Elizabeth tensed waiting for an answer.

"Well, technically he's not your case anymore. Once he had surgery with Dr. Dillon, you signed off so if there were any problems they would have called him."

Elizabeth nodded. "You're absolutely correct." Although she didn't want to, she made a mental note to call him later in the day to follow up on Mr. Byron. Hopefully, she would hear from Caitlyn in the meantime.

"At any rate, here's your schedule of patients for the day. Your first patient is your new best friend, John Martin, aka Lucky."

"How's he doing? We had a shaky start but he seems to be coming around."

"I can tell you he was more respectful today," Heather said with a frown.

"I know he was obnoxious, but I honestly think he was acting out for attention. We'll see. If he straightens out, we'll be fine. If he gets obnoxious again, we'll ask him to leave the practice."

"Well, you can decide when you see him. In the meantime, you've got forty five minutes to work at your desk. He's getting some lab drawn and giving us a urine sample right now."

Nodding, Elizabeth said, "I'll talk to him when he's done. Okay, let me get started here. Thanks Heather. By the way, I bought some fudge for the office. You were right to push me out of here."

"You're welcome. I hope you're feeling better because I'm sure there'll be more charts and messages to come. It is Monday, after all."

One hour later, Elizabeth sat in the exam room with Lucky. "So how am I doing, Doc?"

"I don't have all the lab back, but the few tests they did in the office show improvement. How do you feel?"

Lucky paused for a second. "I think I feel better. I'm less tired and my memory seems better. The only problem is my stomach hurts me sometimes."

Elizabeth nodded. "There's good and bad with everything. Your energy level and memory may be improved because your sugar is more controlled and I'm hoping the lab tests will bear that out. On the other hand, the stomach cramps can be a side effect of eating differently or certain medications at times."

"Yeah, about that, Doc. I feel like a rabbit. I'm dying for a great fast food cheeseburger and fries."

"Lucky, I'm sure I don't even have to go there with you. Diabetics are told to watch their sugar, carbs as well as fat and sodium."

"So what does that leave me? A carrot stick?"

"We had this talk. What that leaves is some nice grilled chicken on top of a nice green salad. You can have eggs and a lot of other veggies and protein."

"Great – that sounds enticing, Doc." Lucky rolled his eyes for emphasis.

"But you're seeing the benefit already. More energy, less fatigue, and sharper brain."

"Maybe I can take those supplements? Maybe that'll help even more?"

"Lucky, why don't we wait a little longer? Supplements are not scrutinized the way other medication is, so we're not positive what effects or even side effects you can have from them. That way, if you do have a problem, we'll know it's more likely from the diabetes instead of the supplements."

Lucky let out a deep sigh. "Okay, you're calling the shots, Doc. So no supplements, donuts, fast food, candy, yada, yada, yada. You're killing me."

"It's the other way around but you're correct in that you can't eat any of the stuff you ate in the past. We'll check your lab every three months or so, for now. Are you walking or exercising?"

"Yes, I walk to the fast food restaurant, look in the window and then walk away after sniffing the aroma, but I'm walking. It's my only mode of transportation."

"Good, I'm glad to hear it, Lucky. You've lost a few pounds and you'll keep going. You'll feel better as each week goes by."

"If you say so."

Elizabeth spent the next fifteen minutes rechecking Lucky's vital signs, examining his heart, lungs, abdomen, eyes and feet. After saying goodbye, she went back to her office and spent another fifteen minutes documenting in his electronic medical record. He could grumble and whine all he wanted as long as he followed his diet. Smiling, Elizabeth knew that Lucky would keep working at it, as long as he knew someone cared about him and the outcome. She requested his next appointment to be scheduled via the recall file.

# CHAPTER 31

Elizabeth spent the rest of the day seeing patients, reviewing charts, fielding phone calls, renewing medications and documenting in the electronic medical record. As she closed out the last note, she realized she hadn't heard from Caitlyn all day.

Bending toward her lower desk drawer, she pulled out her cell phone and checked for messages. Nothing had come in by text or email. Elizabeth sat back in her chair and tried calling her again. When the call went straight to voicemail, she texted a message.

*Hey, where are you? Call me as soon as you can. Even if middle of the night. I need to talk to you.*

SHE TOSSED her phone back into her purse and sat up straight when Heather walked into her office.

"Hi."

Elizabeth looked at Heather and immediately froze.

"What's going on? I don't like that look on your face."

Heather frowned. "You have one more person in the waiting room but he isn't here for a blood pressure check this time."

"Oh no, is it that detective again?"

"Yep, the one and only. Although I still say he's pretty hot," Heather smiled. "Those handcuffs.."

Shaking her head, Elizabeth said, "Can't even imagine, Heather. That's one image I couldn't care less about right now."

"Anyway, he says he wants to talk to you. He asked nicely but it sounds like a long conversation. Can I bring him to your office?"

"Sure, why the hell not? He'll just dog me somewhere else if I don't talk to him. Make sure you send someone with bail money if I get arrested."

"Why would he want to arrest you? Why does he keep coming back?"

"I honestly don't know but it has to do with the death of Frank Burdette."

"Well, then speak with him and get it over with. Maybe he'll give you some information that would help with that other little notice you received."

Elizabeth paused for a moment. "I suppose it wouldn't hurt to see exactly what he wants."

"Okay, I'll bring him in. Then we're all going to leave for the day. I'll text you in fifteen minutes to make sure you're okay. If anything seems strange, text me immediately and I'll connect."

"Thanks, Heather. I appreciate it. By the way, have you heard from Caitlyn recently?"

Shaking her head, she said, "No, I haven't spoken to her in a couple of days."

"Okay, go get him."

"Jake Wagner," Heather said his name dreamily as she turned and headed toward the waiting room.

Elizabeth stayed at her desk. A few minutes later, she heard Heather's voice, "Here you go, Mr. Wagner."

"Thank you," he said. "I appreciate your help."

"You're quite welcome," Heather said. Elizabeth rolled her eyes as she listened to Heather flirt with him. Charm would get him nowhere in her office.

Elizabeth stood up and walked to the door. She pulled the door open to find Heather reaching for the doorknob on the other side.

"Oh, here she is," Heather said.

"Dr. Brooks," Jake said as he extended his hand.

Elizabeth didn't shake hands but stepped back and gestured for Jake to come in. "Thanks, Heather." Raising her eyebrows, she said, "Fifteen minutes, right?"

"Right. Okay, I'll let you go." She gave Jake a small wave from the doorway as she smiled and walked away.

Shaking her head, Elizabeth turned and walked toward her desk. Although there was a conference table in her office, she sat in her desk chair while inviting Jake to sit in one of the seats on the other side.

"How can I help you?" Elizabeth asked.

Jake sat down and crossed his leg. His creased pant leg fell perfectly in line with his Italian shoes. He smiled at her and said, "Look, let's start over. My name is Jake Wagner with the New Wales Police Department. I need your help."

Elizabeth smiled back. "I don't see how I can be of help, but perhaps if you tell me a little more."

There was a knock and Heather opened the door just an inch. "Hi, sorry to interrupt you. We were just leaving and there's a whole bunch of food in the break room and I didn't want to throw it out, especially considering I know the Doc hasn't eaten today," Heather went on in a breathless rush as she walked across the room. "I'm going to put it all on the conference table and then tip-toe out of here. Sorry." Elizabeth and Jake watched in silence as she placed the food on the table and crept out of the room. "Bye, see you tomorrow."

"Is that true?" Jake asked.

"Is what true?"

"Have you had anything to eat today?"

Elizabeth paused. "Now that I think about it, no, I don't think I've eaten since breakfast and that's only because Dr. Covington made me sit and eat. It's not uncommon with medical professionals. We're often too busy to eat or go to the bathroom at times, which I know is completely unhealthy but all too often true. It's a lot of grab and run."

"To be honest, I haven't eaten either. I don't mind moving over to the table and eating while we talk, if that's okay with you." Jake waited for his cue from Elizabeth. He didn't suspect her as part of whatever was going on and wanted to talk to her. Her posture was still defensive at the moment but he hoped it would change.

She looked over at the table and already smelled the delicious aroma of Italian food. "I am hungry. Okay, let's eat."

Jake smiled as he stood and waited for Elizabeth to go first. She set out separating paper plates, utensils and napkins. She then opened the lids of the food containers. Elizabeth always kept an open policy of food in the break room. Meals could not be formalized as the schedule was always fluid so she let the staff order and have food available for whenever they wanted it.

"Nice spread," Jake said as he surveyed the dishes. "You buy lunch every day?"

"Yes, I let them order but they only do that on busy days. To be honest, the restaurant manager is one of my patients so he often throws extra dishes and dessert into the order. Says it keeps him away from the food."

Jake smiled. "That's a good contact to have."

"Yes, especially because he likes to come in and gossip about what goes on in the restaurant."

Jake laughed. "In my business, that's called a CI, confidential informant."

"Hmm," Elizabeth murmured as she handed him a plate. "You have a choice of Cavatelli and Broccoli, Penne with Vodka sauce, Baked Ziti, leftover garlic bread and two slices of pizza. Help yourself."

"Please, you go first," Jake said.

"Alright, let's both dig in. Forget the formality."

"Sounds great to me," Jake said as the pair served themselves from each container and then switched to have a little variety. When their plates were full, they sat near the other end of the table to eat. Elizabeth placed plastic cups in front of them as well as a bottle of water and soda. They sat comfortably for several minutes while they both ate and drank. "I've gotta say, this tastes great. Where do you order from?"

"Carmen's," Elizabeth said after she swallowed. "They're right up the street."

"I'll remember that," Jake said as he broke off a piece of garlic bread. "I hope you don't mind. I'll try not to breathe in your direction."

Elizabeth laughed in spite of herself. "I'm sure garlic breath would not smell any worse than some of the infections I've examined."

"Fair enough," Jake smiled as he popped the last bit of bread in his mouth.

After they both finished their plates and cleaned the crumbs, Jake sat forward with his elbows on the table. Elizabeth's phone started to vibrate with a text.

*Everything okay?*

ELIZABETH TEXTED BACK.

*Yes, I'm fine. Thanks for everything. See you tomorrow.*

*Are you sure? To prove it's you, what's the nickname of your first patient this morning?*

*LOL – Lucky*

*Okay, I'll see you in the A.M. Text me immediately if any problems. Hope the food was good.*

ELIZABETH TEXTED BACK.

*Delicious and necessary. Thanks!*

HEATHER SENT a thumbs-up as her last entry and Elizabeth looked back at Jake.

"Everything okay?"

"Yes, just a last minute message for the office." Elizabeth sat back, took a sip of water and looked at Jake. "Okay, now what's this all about?"

Jake relaxed and appeared to consider where to begin. "I can't discuss the whole case but I want to discuss what I believe is relevant to you."

"Makes sense," Elizabeth said as she waited.

"The department was called in to investigate some irregularities concerning Frank Burdette."

Elizabeth felt an immediate knot in her stomach. "Exactly when was that?"

Jake tried to defuse her tension. "Please relax. We were called in months before his death so it had nothing to do with you. As a matter of fact, I don't believe you're involved in any of this, but I do believe you're going to be able to help me solve this case."

"How so?"

"Let me finish and then we'll explore that."

Elizabeth gestured for him to continue.

"We had an eye on Frank and as I mentioned to you last time, it had something to do with money. During that time, he came to see you as a patient, had surgery and then unfortunately died."

Elizabeth's hands fisted while she listened to him speak.

"Hold on, hear me out," Jake said, sensing the shift. "You understand, we had to follow up, obtain the medical examiner's report and make sure he was dead because it wouldn't be the first time someone had embezzled and skipped the country after faking their death."

Intrigued, Elizabeth relaxed a bit.

"Naturally, when embezzlement is a concern, and I'm trusting you with this information because I'm putting myself on the line here, we then investigate other people in the department and company."

"What company is this?" Elizabeth asked as she wondered just how many other people Jake trusted with information.

"MemorHold. It's a company that makes supplements which they claim will improve your memory and possibly prevent dementia."

Elizabeth knew she had heard the name recently but couldn't remember where.

Jake was gratified to see her initial confusion. "Anyway, within a short time, you examined another patient who worked at MemorHold, a Connie Arturo, and she also died. Surely, you could see our concern."

"Purely coincidental and extremely abnormal as I've never lost a patient before Frank. You well know the cause of death for both of those patient's had nothing to do with the reason they had surgery."

Jake nodded. "So it seems. Are you aware that Randall Byron also worked for MemorHold?"

Elizabeth swallowed as she shook her head. "I hadn't made the connection, but I suppose it would come up if I went through the files."

"So here we are," Jake said with his hands spread out. "I was hoping I could ask you some simple questions about MemorHold and those patients."

"Go ahead and ask, but I don't see how I'm going to be of help. Of course, there is a doctor-patient confidentiality but you appear to know more about my patients than I do at this point."

"Why have you seen three patients from MemorHold in the last six months? Are you related in any way? A company physician?"

Elizabeth shrugged. "I know the company is right down the street because I've seen their sign when I drive to the hospital. It's not uncommon for a company to use the closest hospital system as their preferred provider depending on which insurance they use. My guess would be that was the number one reason, although prior to Frank I had a pretty stellar reputation for surgery and patients."

"So my research has shown," Jake said with a smile.

"Is it odd that three people within the company would all need surgery within a short time?"

Elizabeth shrugged. "I think that would depend on how many people work for the company. If they have ten full time employees and three needed surgery, that would be an awfully high percentage. Now if they have 1000 employees, then no. How big is the company?"

Jake shook his head. "Good question and I don't know."

"So that would be a good place to start," Elizabeth said.

"Do you know or have you ever met Phil Harry?"

"Not that I'm aware of, but I've seen a lot of patients and I don't remember everyone."

"Well, if that were the case, then it wouldn't be significant. I was curious if you personally knew him or contracted to do any specific work for him." Jake watched for her reaction and saw no sign of familiarity with the man or his name.

She shook her head. "His name doesn't sound familiar to me. So I'm still very confused. What exactly is your angle on this?"

"That's my point. I'm trying to find one."

"Well, then let's start over," Elizabeth said. "So there's three people who all work for MemorHold who came to me for surgery and had complications."

"That's correct," Jake nodded. "We're looking into some concerns regarding the company finances and don't know if it's related in any way to the medical issues."

"How could that be? I would understand if I were a plastic surgeon and changed their image, but they're getting their gallbladders and colon cut out. Considering me as part of their conspiracy doesn't make sense."

"I have to agree with you on that one," Jake said. "So then, maybe you have a key to the mystery you don't even realize you have."

Elizabeth shifted in her seat. "Like what?"

"Two of the patients have died. We still have the third patient. Maybe we can talk to him and get some valuable information."

Elizabeth went white at the mention of Mr. Byron.

"What? Why are you making that face?" Jake asked as he watched her pale.

"Ah, we may not have the third patient."

"Why not?"

"Initially, he wasn't doing well. I've been hyper-vigilant since the first two died, so I insisted Mr. Byron have extra testing when he didn't improve. The good news is we did find he was bleeding and the source. I had a vascular surgeon repair his defect and he was coming along. At that point, his care was transferred to Dr. Dillon."

"We can still see him in the hospital, even if I have to do it officially."

"That's the bad news. I went away for a few days and came back last night so I went in early to do rounds at the hospital. When I went to the ICU, he wasn't there."

"Maybe he was moved out to another room."

"I thought that was a possibility, but then I heard a group of residents talking about another surgical ICU death and I kind of freaked. I wasn't able to get details. I tried to reach my friend Caitlyn to fill me in but she hasn't returned my call and I'm a little worried about that too. She always answers my calls."

"Can't you check the hospital computer or something? Wouldn't they have a disposition in his chart?"

Elizabeth nodded sheepishly. "Yes, I could look. I guess I was just too upset to look this morning. I can look now and see if I can find the chart."

"If you wouldn't mind," Jake said. "You'd be helping us out tremendously."

Elizabeth stood and walked to her desk. She turned on her computer and logged in to her medical records. She put Mr. Byron's name into the computer and his chart did surface, with a large notice that she did not have access to his records. "I don't understand this and I don't know why this is happening. They did the same thing with Frank and Connie's charts."

"Who could be blocking you?"

"I have no idea. Sometimes, they'll limit access to a chart as soon as it gets bumped up to risk management in some way."

"Now what?" Jake frowned as he stood behind her at her desk.

Elizabeth shook her head as she furiously continued to tap into the computer. "I don't know. I have to call Caitlyn. She'll know the scoop. I could go into the hospital and start asking questions but that'll raise a whole bunch of red flags especially since Dr. Pruitt," Elizabeth turned to Jake, "he's the Chief of Surgery, has called a meeting to try to get me bounced out of the hospital and yank my license if possible." When Jake didn't respond right away, Elizabeth said, "I trust you won't be spreading that information around or we'll never speak to each other again."

Jake stepped back and crossed his heart. "Not from these lips."

"Good." Elizabeth looked at her watch. "It's getting late. All I can do is try Caitlyn again."

"Where does she live?" Jake asked.

"Why?"

"I'll send a car and an officer to check on her."

"Like hell. She'd never forgive me. She thinks I'm losing it as it is."

"Then I'll go," Jake said. "Give me her address."

"No, you can follow me," Elizabeth said as she stood and put her hands on her hips. "I'll drive over there and you can follow me. I want a chance to explain why the hell I'm dragging a detective over to her place at 7:00 p.m. at night without advanced warning."

"You can't tell her why we're there or any information about the case. We're there to get info, not to offer any." Jake's chiseled face was set, but not unkind.

"I promise," Elizabeth said holding her hand up.

"I have to clear the house first," Jake said, his facial expression indicating he was clearly not tolerating an argument. "Just in case, there's a problem. I'm not sending you into a crime scene or dangerous situation. I shouldn't be having this discussion with you." He rubbed his hands through his hair.

"Fine, I'll drive to her house. Are you following me?"

"Like hell. You're driving me if you won't let me drive." Jake shook his head. "I'm not taking a chance on losing you on our way over. Although you're adorable at times, I'm still wary."

Elizabeth blushed but said sarcastically. "And dinner was so nice."

"C'mon, let's not have our first fight. Grab your keys and let's go. We have to find your patient."

Elizabeth glared at Jake as she reached into her desk drawer and fished out her purse and her keys.

# CHAPTER 32

The pair left Elizabeth's office through the back door and walked out to her car. Elizabeth slipped into the driver's seat as Jake jumped into the passenger's seat. They quickly fastened their seatbelts as Elizabeth started the car. She checked her rear view camera and backed out of her parking space. Navigating onto the highway, she turned left and sped up.

"How far away does she live?" Jake asked while watching the scenery fly by in case he had to retrace the route.

"Not far, about fifteen minutes away. She lives in upper Bergen County."

"What's her last name?" Jake asked.

Elizabeth chuckled. "Always the detective?"

"Just doing my thing," Jake said with a laugh.

"Her name is Caitlyn O'Rourke. She's a float RN but she spends a lot of time in surgical post-op and ICU. She's always been my friend and she's been a great resource for me."

"That sounds like there's a lot more information I shouldn't pry into."

"You've got that right," Elizabeth said as she quickly turned onto another road.

"Hey, Doc. Do you always drive like this?" Jake braced himself on the side door as she completed the turn.

"I do if I'm being summoned to the hospital for emergency surgery."

"I guess that's true," Jake said thoughtfully.

"I tend to get a pass from the local police. They know my car."

Jake chuckled. "I'm sure that's very helpful, and my partner thinks I drive fast."

Elizabeth threw her blinker on and navigated into the left lane. She blew the horn at an oncoming car who was crossing the center line. Jake held the door as he readied for a crash. The oncoming car adjusted into the proper lane and blew past them with his middle finger held high. "Bastard," she said as she slowed the car when they approached a light.

"Next time, I'm driving." Jake complained. "We're not going to do anyone any good if we're dead. I'm glad I didn't decide to follow you."

Elizabeth chuckled as she slowed down and made a left into the driveway of a small ranch home. There was light shining through the living room window in the house. The driveway held one car. Although the sun was setting, Jake could see the lawn wasn't mowed as often as it should have been with weeds popping up around the garden and to the side of the house.

"Is that her car?"

Elizabeth studied the vehicle. "Yes, I'm pretty sure it is. To be honest, I don't see her car because we're always meeting in the hospital."

Jake pulled out his phone and started texting someone.

"What are you doing?"

"I'm texting the plate number to my partner. He'll keep it under wraps but he can run it for information, if need be. He'll also know where to start looking in case anything goes wrong."

"Great, that sounds encouraging," Elizabeth said in a muted voice.

They got out of her car and walked toward the house. Jake put his arm out and motioned for Elizabeth to get behind him. He gestured for her to stay put until he had a chance to check the house. Elizabeth stood in the shadow but jumped when he pulled a gun out of his holster.

Jake cautiously walked toward the house. He looked in the living room window without standing directly in front of it. Elizabeth could tell he didn't see much as he crept from window to window, searching for disaster inside the house.

As Elizabeth watched the bedroom window she saw Caitlyn's outline walking back and forth in front of the shade. The shadow didn't appear to be stressed or harried in any way. Elizabeth walked up behind Jake and tapped him on the shoulder.

He turned to her and put his finger to his lips. Elizabeth rolled her eyes and walked closer to the window. She heard jazz flying through the air, which was a favorite of Caitlyn's. She peeked through the one inch strip of glass that wasn't covered with the shade and she could see Caitlyn walking around the room picking up laundry with one hand and tossing it into a plastic basket. Without hesitating, she reached up and softly knocked on the window.

Caitlyn stopped and looked around, trying to figure out what she just heard. Then Elizabeth knocked again. Caitlyn turned toward the window, fear lining her face. She crept closer and lifted a small amount of shade only to find Elizabeth waving at her through the window. Frowning, she gestured toward the front door.

Elizabeth ran over to the door which was yanked open by her friend. She wore cut off shorts, an old T-shirt and held a beer in her hand. "What the hell are you doing scaring the crap out of me?"

"I'm so sorry," Elizabeth said, just as Jake crept out of the shadows behind her. Caitlyn looked back and forth at Elizabeth and Jake not knowing what to make of the man behind her.

"Are you okay?" Her wide eyes asking if Elizabeth was aware there was a man behind her and if he was nuts.

Elizabeth smiled. "Yes, I'm sorry. Caitlyn, please meet Detective Jake Wagner from the New Wales Police Department." Caitlyn's nod was curt. "Can we come inside and talk with you?"

Caitlyn stepped back and let the pair enter the living room. She smiled when they walked by. "Hello, Jake. Sorry, but you surprised me. Would anyone like a beer?"

They both declined before Elizabeth spoke in a rush. "Where in hell have you been all day? I've been trying to call you for hours. You didn't answer. I thought you were kidnapped or dead."

Caitlyn looked sheepish as she answered. "Oh, my fault completely. I had a whole two days off and I went off the grid. I left my phone in my locker and spent time cleaning the house, sleeping late, drinking beer and screaming at some point. Gotta defervesce as you well know." She giggled as she took a sip of beer.

Elizabeth shook her head. "I asked Heather and she said she didn't know where you were. You always answer your phone."

"Honestly, I was so happy to get a few days off, I flew out of there the minute my shift was over." Caitlyn frowned at Elizabeth. "You just had a few days off so I know you know how it feels."

"Very true and it was wonderful. Almost like a dream, but the minute you return, you're immediately hit with all the stuff you ran away from." As the girls spoke, Jake looked around the room. He took in the worn atmosphere of the furniture, the rug, an out of date television and less than modern kitchen table and chairs. When he heard Elizabeth mention the hospital, he focused back to the conversation.

"Tell me about it. I'm working like crazy to pay off some bills so it's been stressful. What's so important you needed to talk right away?"

Clearing her throat, Elizabeth explained how she went to the hospital this morning to do rounds and check up on Mr. Byron. "I was surprised his bed was empty so I went looking for you and obviously didn't find you so I went to get some coffee." Elizabeth stopped for a deep breath. "Then while I was pouring, the surgical residents were on break and came in talking about another death in the surgical ICU and I kind of freaked out."

"Really? I was hoping you'd relax on your time off."

"I did and I slept better."

"Oh?" Caitlyn asked with a dramatic pause.

Eyes wide, Elizabeth shook her head very subtly so Caitlyn wouldn't say anything about her dreams.

"Yes, and I was able to focus and think about things much more clearly."

"That's great," Caitlyn said, finishing her beer. "So, I'm still confused about what's going on here."

Jake's wrist starting chiming. He turned to read and answer the message he'd just received on his smart watch.

"As much as I hate to talk about it, and I really do, I need to know what happened to Mr. Byron. I can't get into the electronic medical record. You're the only one who can tell me. So I called and texted you and then started worrying about you."

"Okay, well once again, I'm sorry I didn't have my phone. As far as Mr. Byron is concerned, he's probably sleeping right now."

Elizabeth's head snapped up. "What do you mean he's sleeping?"

"I mean he's probably sleeping somewhere. He's coming along, but he's still anemic so I imagine he tires easily."

"Wait, Caitlyn this is important, what about the surgical ICU death?"

She shook her head. "Mr. Byron was transferred to a regular room over the weekend so if someone died in SICU, it wasn't him."

Elizabeth could hardly breathe. "Are you sure? Is there any way you can find out?" Elizabeth spoke rapidly. "Please call someone but don't let them know I want to know."

With raised eyebrows, Caitlyn looked over at Jake who watched quietly. People usually discussed a lot more when they forgot you were in the room. He cleared his throat. "I know Elizabeth is excited, but it's important to find out if Mr. Byron is alive and where he is. He may have some important information for us."

"Okay." Caitlyn went into the kitchen and picked up a cell phone. When Elizabeth stared at her, she said, "This is my very private cell phone number but I'll give it to you as soon as I make a call." As Caitlyn punched in a number, Elizabeth turned to Jake.

"Excited? Really? You've been hawking me and I'm excited? On the other hand, I'll be thrilled if he's alive."

"Don't worry. We're going to find him and talk to him."

"Tonight? Should we be walking into a patient's room late at night to interrogate him?"

"When would you suggest we go? Make an appointment for tea?"

"Don't be a smart ass," Elizabeth said. "My staff and a few hospital employees think I'm nuts already. I don't want to make things worse."

"Listen, if she confirms the patient is alive, we're going to the hospital. Doctors and nurses work with patients day and night."

Elizabeth brushed her hair back from her forehead. "But we have to be quiet. They turn the lights down after 8:00 p.m. so the patients can rest. It is a hospital, after all. Plus, we may have to wake this guy."

"I promise I'll be quiet and discreet," Jake said. "Let's make the contact and we can follow up as needed."

Caitlyn came bouncing into the living room, full of smiles and giggles. "You are never going to believe this." She started to laugh.

"What? Tell me already, what's so funny?"

"Well, it's not funny, but I think you're going to want to hear this."

"Okay, anytime now would be good," Elizabeth said as she thrust her hands on her hips. "Is Mr. Byron alive?"

"Yes, he's definitely alive and he's on third north. Room 3801-2."

Elizabeth hugged Caitlyn. "Thank you. You'll never know how important this was to me." She stepped back. "But then, what's so funny?"

"I'm ashamed to giggle in front of your friend, because it's not funny. Someone in Surgical ICU definitely died and the reason is that he bled out."

"I heard." Elizabeth felt chilled.

Caitlyn nodded. "Yes."

"Then it's happened to someone else. That's terrible for the patient, but validates my claim that something else is going on."

"Here's the part you'll like."

"What? Tell me."

"The surgeon was none other than pissant Pruitt."

Elizabeth stepped back. "Get out, are you sure?"

"Yes, very sure. Apparently, he's been blustering all day. I don't have a name, but the patient was some sort of VIP and attorneys have already requested the records."

"Oh, wow. He must be having a cow. As a matter of fact, he's probably trying to blame me somehow."

"Who knows, but this is big and since it's the third person, you can bet some heads are going to roll. I don't see how the Department of Health doesn't get involved in this."

Elizabeth's stomach tightened as she thought of what the investigation might entail. She turned to Jake. "Listen, we have to keep this controlled. There are a lot of potential implications here for the hospital, the doctors and the patients. It has to be explored but the last thing we want to do is to start a panic." Elizabeth looked at both of them. "We'll go speak to Mr. Byron, but in the meantime, don't talk to anyone else about what's going on. Let's discuss it again tomorrow and decide what to do. I'm sure the hospital will have an opinion as well."

"Okay," Caitlyn said. "I'm working tomorrow. Make sure we catch up."

"We will. I promise," Elizabeth said as she turned to Jake. "If we're going to the hospital, we'd better get going."

The two walked to the front door, followed by Caitlyn. She stopped at the door and watched them walk to Elizabeth's car as she yelled out. "Next time, please try the regular doorbell when you pop in."

Caitlyn giggled to herself thinking Jake was cute. As they pulled out of the driveway, Caitlyn held up her beer in a mock salute.

# CHAPTER 33

Darkness enveloped them as they sped down the Garden State Parkway, trying to get back to the hospital as soon as possible. "I'm glad you're keeping it under 80 mph," Jake said as he watched the lights fly by.

"Okay, okay," Elizabeth laughed. She slowed the car and moved out of the fast lane.

"I appreciate it. As much as I want to get there quickly, I don't want to wind up in the ER as a trauma patient."

"You're no fun," Elizabeth chuckled. They approached the toll and Elizabeth took the right lane EZ Pass in order to keep moving.

Within five minutes, they approached the back parking lot. Elizabeth drove up to the gate, dug her badge out of her purse and waved it at the sensor. They watched the gate open and then drove into the full parking lot, although it was already past visiting hours.

Elizabeth continued to drive through the lot and into the parking garage. She sped around each ramp until she arrived at the fourth level. There she turned into a closed-in area marked, *Physicians Only.* She found an empty stall and parked the car.

Jake looked around. "I hope you park as close to the elevator as possible at night because I'm not sure how safe this is."

"Well, it's not the middle of the night and I'm told there's a security guard who watches very carefully."

Jake turned and frowned at her until she sighed and relented.

"I know there's no safe place if someone wants to get to you but yes, I always try to park as close to the door as I can." Elizabeth picked up her bag.

"Please be careful," Jake said as he unbuckled his seat belt and opened his door. Elizabeth joined him near the elevator but instead of getting on, they walked to a side door which she unlocked with a special digital code. Once the door opened, they walked into a semi-dark room.

Jake watched her, as she turned the lights on and approached the metal cabinets.

When Elizabeth noticed him watching, she explained, "This is the surgical locker room. When clinicians come to work, they wear their street clothes into this room. All personal belongings get locked up and we change into sterile blues before we go into the surgical suite. If I'm making rounds, I store my purse and keys and go into the hall, which is exactly what we're going to do now."

Jake nodded and scanned the room, taking it all in. Elizabeth closed the locker door and beckoned for Jake to follow her. She pushed open a heavy oak door into the main hallway. As they stepped through, Jake heard the door click shut behind them. He turned back and noticed the digital lock before he heard Elizabeth call. "C'mon, it's getting late." She was looking at her phone. "I'm checking admissions to confirm the room number. After pressing the screen several times, she tapped Jake on the arm. "I found him. He's on the third floor just like Caitlyn said. I'm so happy he's alive."

"I can see that."

"C'mon, let's go." Elizabeth walked ahead of him, eager to find her patient well and in good hands. They walked through the darkened halls, indicating visiting hours were over for the day. A quiet hush reverberated through the area. Nurses were busy behind the desk or working with medication carts in the hall. Some were walking into rooms to deliver medications, take vitals and check wounds. Machines beeped while call buttons rang.

The only other time Elizabeth felt a similar hush was while sitting in an empty church. Despite a lack of activity, the air contained an expectant energy which was only dispelled when normal activity began.

They reached the door and Elizabeth peered inside. Mr. Byron was lying in the bed, watching television. Elizabeth let out a sigh of relief when she realized the bed next to him was empty. She didn't want anyone to witness the patient being questioned by the police this late at night but she also didn't want to approach him during the day. With her luck, someone would call the Risk Management Department the minute she asked the first question. The room was relatively dark, the only light being the one over the bed which pointed toward the ceiling. The bed was semi-upright with the tray table nearby. On the table she spied a plastic water pitcher, cups, a cell phone, one get well card and a newspaper crossword puzzle.

Elizabeth turned to Jake and waved for him to follow her into the room. She gently knocked as they crossed the threshold and smiled when Mr. Byron looked up at them.

"Hi, Randall. I know it's late. You up for some company?"

"Hey, Doctor Brooks. I'm glad to see you."

"I'm glad to see you, too. How are you feeling?" Elizabeth walked to the bedside and Jake followed along behind her.

Randall tried to sit up but shifted awkwardly, as pain shot through his side. "Well, I'm much better now that I'm in a regular room. I don't know what the hell happened back there. I think I remember you saying the surgery was over but then it was all a blur. I felt like I was in a dream for a week. Hell, I don't even remember going back for the second surgery, but the vascular surgeon did a great job and I felt better within a day or so."

Elizabeth's heart sunk as Randall Byron answered her questions. "Well, I'm certainly glad you're feeling better."

"Thanks to you," he said as he beamed.

"Me?"

"Oh, yes. Dr. Dillon said he never would have operated if you didn't insist but you were right. Thanks to you, I'm still here."

Elizabeth smiled at his words. Maybe Caitlyn was right that she was harder on herself than she needed to be. "Well, it's interesting you say that. One of the reasons I'm here tonight is to talk about what happened." Elizabeth pulled over the bedside chair and spoke in a very soft voice as she sat down. "I've brought a…," she looked up at Jake. "A colleague with me to talk about your health."

"Okay, I feel bad that you have to keep such late hours but I can't sleep anyway, so that's fine."

"Great," Elizabeth said, relieved he had agreed to talk this late at night. "You know, before your surgery, I reviewed all of your medical records. I looked at your medications and past surgeries. So, I'm a little confused about what happened. After the first surgery, you started bleeding. More than you should have and you weren't bleeding near the surgical site."

"I know, Dr. Dillon said I basically burst a vessel near my kidney."

"Yes, that's right," Elizabeth said. "My colleague and I are trying to figure out if you have any risk factors for having a vessel burst."

Randall shook his head. "I have no clue. No one in my family ever had a problem like that so it makes no sense to me."

Jake moved toward the bed and looked at Mr. Byron. "Mind if I ask a few questions?"

"I've got nothing to hide." Randall lifted an eyebrow and shrugged.

"Thanks," Jake said as he shook his head. "My name is Jake, by the way."

"Nice to meet ya, Jake." The two men shook hands.

"One of the reasons I asked Dr. Brooks to allow me to talk to you is because we're concerned about deaths in the hospital and the community. I have to be honest with you, I'm a detective with the New Wales Police Department."

"The police department? What's going on?"

"That's what we're trying to find out. Do you know a man named Frank Burdette? Or a woman by the name of Connie Arturo?"

"Of course I do. I work with both of them on occasion," Randall said. "They're in a completely different division so I haven't seen them in a long time."

Jake nodded and looked at Elizabeth who took over. "Randall, I can't say much because of confidentiality laws, but what I can say is that we are seeing a small trend of problems with patients who work at MemorHold, so I was wondering if there was anything different about where you work or what you may do there."

Randall thought for a moment and shrugged. "Nothing I can think of."

Jake leaned forward again. "Can you take us through a typical day at your job? We don't know for sure if there's a problem, but we're trying to rule out any common exposures for anyone with a problem. For example, if fifteen people who eat at the same restaurant get sick on the same night, we go in and check the restaurant."

Randall nodded. "I see what you're getting at, but I feel bad. I didn't know Frank or Connie had a problem. I'll have to reach out to them."

Elizabeth shot Jake a warning look and he frowned back at her.

"Let's see. I go to work around 9:00 a.m. each morning." Randall looked up at Elizabeth. "I work in supplies so there's nothing exciting going on over there. I go to work, check the requests and fill them. Mostly, it's internal need. If a manager needs folders, a calendar, or even a pen, I run it over."

Elizabeth nodded while she thought. "What about chemicals or anything that would be considered a biohazard? Do you handle anything like that?"

Randall laughed. "No, I don't think so. Jeez, even the correction fluid is now a tiny strip of plastic. Nothing with those little bottles people can sniff. Besides, we have to keep the plant as clean and sterile as possible since we make supplements. The staff who work near the pill room have to wear those little green hair nets like you stuck on me right before surgery."

Elizabeth chuckled. "You know they're at the height of fashion."

"Apparently," Randall said, playing along. "I guess that's why they wear them at the plant."

"Do you ever go near the supplements?"

"Not in the area where they're being bottled, but I have gone into the distribution area."

Perplexed, Elizabeth asked, "And what happens there?"

"That's where all the bottles are boxed, sealed and shipped to whomever ordered them. They have the free bottles there as well."

Elizabeth shook her head. "I'm sorry, I don't understand. Tell me about the free bottles."

Randall nodded as he spoke. "Some of the bottles are slightly irregular or the lids are cracked, but the supplements are okay. They put those in a bin for employees to take. It's like working for a candy factory, you always see big bowls of candy except at MemorHold it's supplements for your memory. To be honest, I'd rather be working in the candy factory."

Elizabeth looked at Jake who raised his eyebrows. "Excuse me, Randall. Do they put any limits on who can take these supplements or what you can do with them?"

"Of course, we're told never to sell them and we can only take two bottles per month, but honestly, no one monitors that."

"So, if someone wanted, say ten bottles for their family at home, they'd have access to it?"

Randall slowly nodded his head, unasked questions fleeting across his face. He was suddenly wary of answering any further questions.

"I'm not sure what this has to do with my operation but I think I'm starting to get tired."

Elizabeth stood up. "I understand. It's getting late and we appreciate being able to spend some time with you. I'm sorry if we kept you up."

"No, it's fine," Randall said. "I hope I helped you."

"You did. Thank you, Randall," Elizabeth said as she smiled. Jake leaned forward and shook his hand.

"Sleep well, I hope you're out of here soon."

"I hope so too. Doc, I'll come see you in the office when I'm due for a follow up."

"Sounds good, Randall. See you then."

Elizabeth and Jake turned and left the hospital room. Elizabeth put her finger to her lips to let Jake know he should be quiet. They made their way down several dark corridors until they reached the door for the surgical locker room. Elizabeth punched in a code and the door shifted with a large click. Pulling the door open, they walked inside and stopped at Elizabeth's locker. After retrieving her purse and keys, they slipped out the back to Elizabeth's car.

After putting on their seat belts, Elizabeth started the car and drove out from the parking deck. "Okay, so now what?"

"I think it's time to visit MemorHold and meet the CEO," Jake said quietly as he settled back into his seat.

# CHAPTER 34

It took fifteen minutes for them to reach her office. Elizabeth parked the car and turned to Jake. "It's been an interesting day, but I have to go home."

"Got it," Jake said. "Thanks for taking the time to help me out. You went above and beyond with your friends and contacts today. You even fed me first."

"You should be thanking Heather, not me," Elizabeth said.

"Next meal is on me." Jake smiled as he unlatched his seat beat. "Criminals I'm good with, but what's the next step if this supplement is a problem?"

"Usually, a person would go to the portal for the FDA and report it. It's a little different with a supplement than a prescription medication, but they'll still investigate it. Depending on the complaint, evidence presented and initial investigation, they'll follow it as long as they have to."

"Would they shut them down?"

"Yes, if it poses enough of a serious danger. They would issue a recall and then issue a notice to the media to notify the public."

"So, the CEO would have a lot to lose," Jake nodded.

"Potentially, his company, his job, his reputation, as well as face a class action lawsuit, but it doesn't necessarily mean he did anything criminal," Elizabeth explained. "Now, if they can prove he knew there was a problem, but continued to market, advertise and put the public in danger, he'd be in a heap of trouble."

"Will you be calling the FDA?" Jake asked as he watched her profile.

Elizabeth shook her head. "Not yet, you have to give something credible. There's not enough evidence of a medical problem. I need to look into a few things and then I'll decide. What about the criminal part?"

"I have to call my partner," Jake said.

"Adam?" Elizabeth asked.

Jake chuckled. "No, his name is Alex Houghton. He's been texting me on and off since I sent that license plate to make sure we don't need to call in the troops. I'll call him as soon as I'm in my own car."

"Sounds good," Elizabeth said, the situation now getting awkward.

"Are you going back into the office?" Jake asked. "If you are, I'd like to wait long enough to make sure you get your things and get back to your car safely."

Elizabeth paused. "Well, yes I do have to go back in, but I won't be long and now that you offer, I'd appreciate it. Sometimes, it's a bit creepy when it's dark. There's no security guard here."

"Tonight, you have me. Okay, let's get to it," Jake said. The awkward moment over, the two got out of Elizabeth's car and walked toward the back entrance of the office. Elizabeth dug out her keys and opened the back door. Stepping in front of her keypad, Elizabeth punched in her code and turned off the alarm. She went into her office and quickly went through the papers on her desk. Jake patiently waited while she checked her appointments for the next day and made sure she had the schedule clear in her mind. Elizabeth smiled at Jake as she grabbed her things and they headed for the back door.

Once everything was locked up, Jake walked Elizabeth to her car and held the door as she slid into the driver's seat.

"Thanks, again," Elizabeth said. "I appreciate you staying."

"It's the least I could do since you helped so much," Jake said. He hesitated before he closed her driver's door. "You know, I'll probably have to talk to you about the case so I hope it's okay if I call you."

Elizabeth immediately felt butterflies in her stomach as they exchanged cell numbers. "Sure, normally I wouldn't do this because I strongly believe in patient confidentiality, but there's more here than meets the eye and to be honest, it's in my best interest to get to the truth." Not knowing why, Elizabeth's face reddened and she looked down at her lap.

Jake nodded. "I understand. I'll talk to you soon. You'd better get going."

Elizabeth started the car, closed the window and pulled out of the parking lot.

# CHAPTER 35

Elizabeth arrived home and hurried into the condo. It was late and she needed to accomplish a few things before she went to bed. Although she normally wasn't as paranoid, she made sure all the doors and windows were securely locked for the night. Perhaps that's what happens to someone when they hang around with a detective for a few hours. Elizabeth felt her face flush when she thought of Jake. He was incredibly handsome but she reminded herself he was a detective trying to solve his case. Nothing more.

The answering machine was blinking but she went through her mail and placed her things on the hall desk before she checked her messages. As she went to hit the button, the desk phone rang, making her jump at the sound. Elizabeth picked it up, expecting to hear the voice of someone from her answering service.

"Elizabeth? Is that you? Are you there?"

"Mom?" Elizabeth was confused when she heard her mom's voice. "Is everything okay?"

"That's what I wanted to ask you. I've been calling you for hours. Then I got worried when you didn't answer your cell or your phone and I couldn't reach you."

"My cell didn't ring," Elizabeth said as she dug into her purse and pulled her cell phone out. She had been grateful she didn't have to deal with any office calls while she was with Jake but now she was anxious when she realized the phone silence was longer than unusual. She looked at the phone and noticed it wasn't on. She pushed the button with no response. How could the phone have died? She felt bad she had complained to Caitlyn about the very same thing. "Hold on, Mom," she said as she pulled out a charger and quickly plugged it in.

"Mom, my cell phone was dead, but I didn't realize it. I plugged it in to charge and I'll have to wait a few minutes to check it. Is everything okay? Why were you calling?"

"I wanted to check on you. You were so upset this weekend and I know you went back to work today so I wanted to make sure everything was okay. Things are easier when you're away from the source of the stress but it's hard to jump back into the mouth of the dragon. Believe me, I know. Your father and I had to go through our share of that throughout our life."

Elizabeth was quiet as she considered her mother's words. She watched as her phone generated a small charge and then noticed several text messages and missed calls pop through. "Here they all come, now."

"Anyway, is everything okay? Usually, you're home much earlier. Why were you out so late?"

Elizabeth didn't know what to say. She didn't want to tell her mother about Jake and the investigation over the phone but she could stretch the truth a bit. "I went into work this morning and checked on my last surgical patient but I couldn't find him. To be honest, I got upset because I thought he died. After office hours, I went to see Caitlyn and she told me he had been moved to another room so I went back to the hospital to chat with him. Thankfully he's okay. I'd be devastated to find out there was another death."

"I'm glad he was okay."

There was a pause for a few moments which prompted Elizabeth to ask. "Mom, are you sure you're okay?"

"Yes, yes, I'm fine and your father's fine as well. As a matter of fact, he's been talking to John Donovan all day. He wants to help you solve this as soon as possible."

"That's sweet," Elizabeth said as she smiled. She missed being with her parents more than she thought.

"I'm worried," her mother said with a sigh. "I'm upset this has started over again and you felt the need to escape."

"I know, Mom. In the beginning I was panicking, but I received some new information today that may work out in my favor. The police are looking into it and hopefully I'll know something soon."

"I hope so, dear. Your father may have something for you, too."

"I'll be calling him in a day or two and then he can fill me in," Elizabeth said. "I just got home and need to do a few things to be ready for tomorrow but I'll call soon. I promise. Please tell him. Also let him know I'll be dropping the records off at the post office tomorrow."

"I will, Dear. It may be better if you come down and discuss it. Goldy has been pouting ever since you left. It's amazing. We took the dog in, have fed and cared for her but from the minute she met you, she's been obsessed with you. She stared out the window all day looking for you."

"Aww, she's so sweet. I promise I'll try to come back soon. She's quite a dog."

"Yes she is. I'll let you go as long as you're okay. Please stay in touch and let us know what's going on."

"Will do, Mom. Love you."

"Love you more."

"Goodnight," Elizabeth said as she hung up the phone. She hadn't seen her parents in a while and knew she purposely stayed away after all the pain her dreams had caused them. Countless medical exams, appointments for tests and meetings with psychiatrists and neurologists, Elizabeth could understand why no one wanted to open that black hole again. She was sure the stress of the last couple months had something to do with it. She'd sort it all out one day, but not tonight and not right now. Elizabeth wanted to settle down and go to bed. Her routine was off and she instinctively knew that when her eating, sleeping and self care were off, things happened. Sometimes, bad things.

# CHAPTER 36

Elizabeth pulled back the comforter and got ready to slip into bed. She was looking forward to being surrounded by cool, soft material and relaxing after a hectic, yet hopeful day. When Frank died, she thought her career, her professional life as she knew it, was over. The lawsuit certainly didn't help either. Elizabeth had gone to her parents trying to plan what she would do with the rest of her life, after she dealt with the shame and needless guilt of killing several patients. She didn't believe she had done anything wrong but the patients had died. Maybe there was hope after today. Elizabeth turned on her side and drifted off to sleep.

She did well for most of the night, but toward early morning, she began to moan and twitch as she fell into a deeper REM sleep.

*ELIZABETH WALKED along the path and Frank waited for her. He was up ahead and there were a lot of people standing behind him. She stood where she was and looked at him with questioning eyes. He waved her on. "C'mon, you gotta keep going. You finally started on the right path, but you got a ways to go yet and you're not out of danger. Keep going."*

*She looked at him and seemed to be asking him a question without speak-*

*ing. Perhaps he could read her mind because he answered her. "I know you don't have all the answers yet, but they're gonna start coming to you real soon. There's a lot of people back here who wanted to tell you directly, but I convinced them to let me be the spokesperson so we don't scare you out of your mind. A lot of people got hurt, you have to do something about it. Keep going. There's more than you think."*

ELIZABETH'S EYES BLINKED OPEN. It took her a few moments to realize where she was and that she was safe. Her breathing and heart rate were more rapid than usual but nowhere near as fast as they were in the past when she dreamed. She still had no idea what Frank was trying to tell her, but she knew she was on the right track. Jake felt it too and together they were getting somewhere. Now, she just had to stay on the trail. Jake said he would call her but if he didn't, she'd call him. She had to get to the truth before it was too late.

Elizabeth rolled onto her other side. She now faced her side table and reached for a pad and a pen. Sitting up slightly, and with just a hint of light through the window, she wrote down everything she remembered about her dream. One of her early counselors, suggested years ago that she write down her dreams to see if they could identify a cause or a meaning. She'd forgotten as it was something she hadn't done in years, but it all came flooding back so easily now.

She wrote down the specifics as well as she could and then allowed herself to release the image, the thoughts, the anxiety and drift back to sleep. Elizabeth had another two hours before she had to get up and go to work. She needed the rest.

# CHAPTER 37

Elizabeth woke early and got ready for work. She wanted to race to the hospital, find Caitlyn and tell her about Jake. She could envision her now, either rolling her eyes at the story or yelling at her for sneaking up the night before.

She parked in the lot, hurried inside, threw her things in her locker and headed toward the surgical ICU. Checking the census, she made sure none of the patients were hers. She hadn't performed any procedures in the last six days, but she was scheduled for surgery on Thursday.

Looking around the desk, she found the nurses's assignments and Caitlyn's name listed as the nurse for the last three cubicles. Elizabeth discreetly put the clipboard back where it belonged and headed to the corner of the ICU.

She spotted Caitlyn hanging an IV over an elderly man. He looked very frail and Elizabeth watched as Caitlyn plugged in his medicines with utmost confidence and respect. Elizabeth had never met this man but he tugged on her heart strings. Some patients were so weak, so frail and so trusting that it pained her not everyone could be saved.

Elizabeth waited in the small area outside the cubicle until Caitlyn emerged. "Good morning."

"Oh, I didn't see you out here."

"I wanted to wait until you were done. That poor guy looks so weak."

"He is but he's a cute little guy. He's here for an infection and heart problems. I just hung an antibiotic and hopefully it'll kick in soon."

Elizabeth pulled her to the side. "I have to talk to you."

Caitlyn grinned. "Yes, I'd like to talk to you, too. That was some hottie you were with last night. Nice suit he was wearing."

"Stop it. We're only following up on a case."

Caitlyn burst out laughing. "A case? Have you been undercover as a detective or surgeon all this time?"

Elizabeth rolled her eyes. "Seriously, you have to help me. You ripped into me last week and told me to get my shit together so here I am, putting my life back together. Now help me out with something."

Caitlyn sighed and put her hands on her hips. "Outside the ICU. Let's go talk."

"Great. I want you to try to do something for me and then we can get a cup of coffee at the café."

Caitlyn looked at her watch. "I need ten minutes before I go on break. Why don't you get our coffee and meet me in the chairs by the window. No one ever goes there so we should have privacy."

"You've got it," Elizabeth said. "Make sure you come. I'm dying to talk to you."

"Evidently," Caitlyn frowned. "Go and let me finish this med pass so I can leave."

Elizabeth turned and left the ICU, urgency etched in her eyes.

Twelve minutes later, Caitlyn joined her in the lounge. Her coffee was waiting on a side table. She picked it up and looked at the cup as she took her first sip.

"Heavenly," Caitlyn said. "Which should indicate just how badly I need coffee. Ok, shoot. What's the emergency?"

"I'm not sure, but we may have made a small break in the case," Elizabeth said and then held her hand up as Caitlyn began to smirk again. "Just listen to what I have to say. I'm not supposed to talk to anyone but I need you to do something."

"Of course," Caitlyn said dryly.

"Now don't be that way," Elizabeth said.

"I'm not," Caitlyn said. "I told you I'd help you however I could. So what do you want me to do?"

Elizabeth leaned forward to speak in a conspiratorial whisper. "The one thing Jake said when he came to speak with me yesterday, was that the two patients who died after surgery both worked at MemorHold. He got pulled into this investigation because of some problem with their finances, but the medical part is completely random. When we spoke to Randall last night, and yes we did find him, he also talked about MemorHold. He knew of Frank and Connie but hadn't seen them in a long time and didn't know they were dead. So when we questioned him at length, he mentioned there was a bin full of supplements at MemorHold for workers. However, the usage is not monitored and there's no follow up. Randall didn't admit to taking their supplement on a regular basis, and when he realized we were asking a lot of questions, he clammed up real fast. But, he told us enough to start looking into whether there's a connection to MemorHold for all the dying patients."

"Oh snap," Caitlyn said. "So what do you want me to do?"

Although Caitlyn didn't think it was possible, Elizabeth drew even closer. "You mentioned that the last patient who died in Surgical ICU was a patient of pissant Pruitt, right?"

"Yes, can you believe it? The poor man died and Pruitt was incensed. The family was there, in the cubicle. They were devastated and Pruitt has the nerve to be pissed off. Forget about compassion and empathy. I heard he was ticked off and blaming this man for being a blemish on his record. I can't believe it. What a complete ass."

"Wow," Elizabeth said. "I can't say I'm shocked, but I'm pretty disgusted."

"You, me, and every other person in the ICU. So, what do you want me to do?"

"Obviously, I can't go into the medical record. IT monitors everything, but since you were a nurse taking care of him, you'd have access to that chart."

"Yes, but that chart is already flagged so I can't just run through it."

"I don't want you to. I just want you to get a medication list and his pre-op history and physical. I want to know if he worked for Memor-Hold or took any of their supplements. That's all I need to know. I don't care about Pruitt's surgical technique and that's the area that will be most protected. Just tell them you want to check your documentation, that's all."

Caitlyn sighed and frowned at Elizabeth. "You're lucky they haven't locked it down yet. As a matter of fact, they want to make sure all notes are complete so I'll probably be able to do it, but just for the record, I'm not in the habit of doing things that may cost me my license."

"I know and I swear I'll never ask you to do something like this again." Elizabeth pleaded with her eyes. "Please."

Caitlyn chugged down the rest of her coffee and put the mug on the table near her. "I'll see what I can do. Don't call me. I'll text or call you when I can."

Elizabeth was thrilled and wrapped her arms around her friend in a bear hug. "Don't text me any details. At most, just use a yes or no and I'll know what it means. I'll ask you plenty of specific questions when I see you."

Caitlyn stood up, shook her head and got ready to leave. She looked back at Elizabeth and said, "You owe me."

# CHAPTER 38

"Jake Wagner." He sat at his desk and picked up the phone on the second ring. He listened to someone speak for several minutes before answering. "Thanks, I appreciate it. I'll let you know."

"What's going on?" Alex asked as Jake hung up the phone.

"One of my buddies at the DEA. I called to see if Phil Harry is a common name around their department. He didn't recognize it so he said he'd do a little digging."

"And?" Alex asked, frowning.

"DEA apparently doesn't have him on a watch list, but that's because he doesn't deal with any meds that are narcotics or scheduled. He reached out to his buddies, but nothing yet. He told me to try the FDA and possibly Better Business Bureau."

"I can tell you there's nothing official out there," Alex said. "I would know, being the master of the internet, dark web and otherwise." Alex preened. "You'd probably get more info by checking out his social media accounts."

Jake smiled. "Hey, don't laugh. Sometimes it's a detective's best friend."

"Anyway, while you were out playing last night, I did gather some information." Alex took on a serious tone, picked up a cup of cold coffee and gulped it down.

"I wasn't out playing. I was working with a confidential informant, a new CI."

"So I'm told. What did you and your new CI come up with, so to speak?" Alex frowned when Jake smiled.

"You son of a bitch."

"No, nothing happened. Not even close. I have to ask permission just to call and ask her a question about the investigation. As honored as I am that you think my charm is so irresistible, that's one avenue that's blocked for me."

"Good, and I hope it's killing you," Alex said as he threw a crumpled piece of paper at Jake's head. "So, did you get any info or not?"

Jake nodded as he typed into his computer. "She took me to a recent surgical patient who had complications. It was the third patient with problems and the guy confirmed he worked for MemorHold. Interestingly, he told us there's a bin with samples for the workers to take home. They're probably rejects according to quality control or have a little something extra in them for the employees."

"Really?"

"Yeah, after a while he stopped talking because he realized he was getting into some deep water. The question is, What exactly is the boss handing out to his employees? It sure doesn't seem like it's helping them. Apparently, the guy knew our other players but didn't see them too often. As a matter of fact, if you believed him, he didn't know they were dead."

"So the primary connection is where they work, not in their relationship."

"Seems so," Jake said as he hit send on the computer and turned toward Alex. "We need to know more about our CEO."

Alex picked up a sheaf of papers and handed Jake a photograph of a early, middle-aged, good looking gentlemen. "Phil Harry, forty-eight year old pharmaceutical executive. His bio says he's had twenty-four years of experience in the pharmaceutical field. Started as a rep for one of the big Pharma companies and eventually worked his way up in a few start-ups. To be honest, he looks like the type of guy who would kiss his boss's ass in order to get a promotion." Jake chuckled as he listened. "Most of the start-ups he was affiliated with closed down within six months except for his latest, MemorHold. The paperwork lists the product as the supplement with the same name, MemorHold which is purported to help prevent memory loss. There may be a few other products sold by the company, related to dementia."

"Like what?" Jake asked as he scribbled on paper.

"Let's see, tactile blankets, orientation calendars and clocks, journals for memoirs, books for caregivers and other things along that line."

"Fancy," Jake said. "Does he have sales? Credibility? Where does the company stand?"

Alex nodded. "Like they always say, follow the money. It seems this company has a couple of anonymous investors who provided enough of a cash flow to make his first year profits look legitimate, but since then, the company appears to be losing a lot of money or making it disappear somewhere else."

"What about sales? Is there any way you can track whether he's making any?"

"I don't have concrete numbers on that. He's put some money toward advertising and there's a long list of local pharmacies that have stocked their shelves with his supplement but it's a long road to reach the national familiarity of most meds or vitamins. Most of these small companies try to develop a solid sales record and then sell their whole company to a national chain for a decent profit, often in the millions."

"In the meantime, we should check to see how many complaints came in about the drug especially if it's been out there awhile."

"What about the FDA?"

"I'm going to let the good doctor look into that for the moment. She'll be able to research some things better than me and supply more convincing information to pull in investigators."

"And I'm sure you'll have to meet frequently to discuss her progress," Alex said as he rolled his eyes.

"These things do need to be monitored appropriately," Jake said with a small laugh.

"I swear, you're an ass."

"Listen, it's not like that with Elizabeth."

"We're on a first name basis?"

"Well, we spent the night breaking into her girlfriend's house and then running to the hospital after hours. I couldn't keep calling her Dr. Brooks."

Alex shook his head as he went back to typing on his keyboard. "So what next?"

"We need to talk to Connie's girlfriend and see what she knows about the company. We specifically need to ask about that bin of samples. After that, I think it's time we go visit Mr. Harry and ask him about his employees. Something stinks with this whole case and it's time to get to the truth."

# CHAPTER 39

Elizabeth left the cafe and checked on Mr. Byron. She didn't go into the room as she didn't want to bother him, but she checked to make sure he was healing well and had discharge planning in place. If she had her way, she would have put a bodyguard on the man.

Once she was satisfied he was safe, she left the hospital and went back to the office. She went in through the back door and placed her things on her desk. Sensing someone was in the hall, Elizabeth opened the door to find Heather on the other side, poised to knock. Heather pulled her fist back when she saw Elizabeth.

"Hey, I was just coming to check on you," Heather said. "To be honest, I drove by last night when I went out with one of my friends and your car was gone but the detective's car was still in the parking lot. I noticed his car was gone this morning so there must be some interesting information you can share." Heather wasn't sure if she should be sporting a smug expression or not.

"Not like that, Heather. Calm down," Elizabeth said with a shake of her head. "We found Caitlyn at home and she helped answer some questions about problems at the hospital. We drove there together."

"Really? What's going on?" Heather asked. "There's been a lot of angst."

Elizabeth paused, not sure what to say. She pulled Heather into the room and sat her down at the conference table. When she was settled, Elizabeth began, "There's been a lot of weird things going on with patients and surgeries and there's an investigation to see if we can find out why."

Heather nodded as if she understood completely. "Okay, I'm not exactly sure what you're looking for but I get it."

"I'll tell you what I'm looking for. When you get time, I want you to sort through as many medical records as possible and look at the medication lists. I want to know if any of our patients are taking a supplement called MemorHold."

Heather thought for a moment. "Isn't that the one your favorite patient, Lucky, keeps asking about?"

"You know, you're right," Elizabeth said. "But, as I recall, I told him to hold off so we know if the diabetes gives him any side effects. I don't like to start several new things at once."

"Let's hope he listens," Heather said with a side nod of her head.

"Well, that's the point. If Lucky knows about it, then probably everyone in the same circle knows about MemorHold. Please go through the charts and med lists and give me the name of every patient who is or was on it. I need to reach out and see if there are problems."

"You've got it, boss," Heather said. "I put all your messages on your desk. There were a couple of repeats from last night."

"My fault completely. I didn't get to all the calls, but as I recall none of them were emergencies."

"No, but they called back today and they're still waiting on you."

"I get it," Elizabeth said. "I will not leave the office today until I finish every single one."

"Okay, I'm depending on you because I don't want to hear from them again tomorrow."

"You shouldn't. In the meantime, I have surgery scheduled tomorrow morning?"

"Yes, I'll hand you all the prep sheets after your first couple of patients."

"Thanks, Heather. I appreciate it so much."

"You're welcome," Heather smiled. "I'm glad we got to meet that cute detective at any rate."

"Well, don't expect him to be hanging around too often. Once he gets what he needs, he'll be gone."

Heather shrugged and sported an evil grin. "I don't know, maybe his blood pressure will act up again."

Elizabeth rolled her eyes and pointed toward the hall. Just as Heather was about to leave, Elizabeth called her back. "Do me a favor. Please reach out to Lucky this morning. See if he's okay. Ask him if he's taking that supplement."

"I thought you told him not to," Heather said.

"Since when do patients listen to their doctor?" Elizabeth asked sporting a frown.

Heather nodded. "Gotcha, I'll call him right away."

# CHAPTER 40

"Phil Harry, please." Jake managed to command more than ask to see the man. The administrative assistant sat at the desk, unmoving. She was well dressed, sitting ramrod straight, with ankles crossed and black stilettos on her feet. Jake often wondered how women spent the whole day in stilettos without suffering back pain.

"He's on a conference call at the moment. Is he expecting you?"

"Not really, but we'll be happy to wait," Jake said with a large smile, charm flowing from his eyes. She stared up at his face, then smiled a bit.

Alex turned away so she wouldn't see him frown.

"And your name is?" She asked.

"Jake Wagner and my partner is Alex Houghton."

She tilted her head and flirted as she asked. "Can I have the name and number of your firm?"

Jake smiled. "How about I leave that info on the way out? Maybe a little more as well?"

The woman blushed and looked down at her phone. "Perhaps he's off his call. Let me check." Using an intercom, she buzzed her boss and turned her chair so her back was facing them. Jake could hear her whisper that two gentlemen were here to see him and had been waiting. He asked questions which she deflected expertly. "Yes sir," she said and hung up the phone.

She turned back to find Jake smiling at her, while Alex had given up and taken a seat near the wall. She smoothed her hair and said, "He'll see you. I'll bring you back in a moment."

"Great," Jake said as he reached over and straightened the pens and pencils on the assistant's desk.

A moment later, she received a buzz on her phone. "I'll take you back now."

She stood up and managed to lead the two men to a large office in the back. Pivoting on her skinny heel, she smiled at Jake as she backed out of the room and pulled the door closed after her.

Plush carpeting covered the floor. A large glass desk sat in the corner with leather chairs set across. Floor to ceiling windows looked over a garden filled with rocks and flowers. A large couch was sitting against the side wall. Jake had to wonder if the administrative assistant had ever observed the ceiling from that piece of furniture.

"Please have a seat. How can I help you gentlemen?" Phil Harry settled back into his desk chair. Jake watched him as he moved. Phil was athletic, slim, and filled out his expensive suit. He had a decent head of hair for a 48 year old. His demeanor was arrogant as if their mere presence was wasting his precious time. He shot his cuffs and looked at the two of them expectantly.

"Thank you for seeing us, Mr. Harry." Jake reached out to shake his hand. "I'm Detective Wagner with the New Wales Police Department and this is my partner Alex Houghton."

"Police Department?" Phil said as his head snapped up. "What's this all about?"

Jake wanted to draw Phil out without scaring him off. "We're here to talk to you about Frank Burdette and Connie Arturo. They were former employees."

"Yes, they were. Very tragic what happened to them," Phil said in a smooth polished voice reserved for these type of discussions. "Are you investigating that quack doctor who operated and killed them? It would be great to get her off the street. Who knows how many other lives you may save?"

Although he didn't let it show, Jake was surprised to feel his anger rise. He cleared his throat before he spoke. "We're trying to look at everything, Mr. Harry, which is why we're here to ask you a few questions."

"Well, I don't know what I can tell you, but I have a few minutes," Phil said without much expression as he made it a point to look at his Rolex.

Jake cleared his throat to refocus Phil's attention and began. "We wanted to know a bit more about the employees. What can you tell us about Frank Burdette?"

Phil thought for a few minutes. "I don't know much about him. I don't have time to fraternize with the staff. He seemed like a nice guy. I think he had a wife and some kids, but not totally sure about that."

Alex interrupted. "I thought you went to services or acknowledged them after the death."

"I'm sure I did or sent flowers or something, but I can't remember everything about the staff. It's a shame but I'm sure they'll be fine with whatever life insurance he had."

Jake grew irritated. "What about his position here? I believe we were told he was an accountant. How was his work performance?"

Phil stiffened at the question. "I suppose it was fine as he wasn't fired or put on leave." Phil looked directly at Jake. "How did you say this investigation got started?"

"I didn't, really. It's just that two seemingly healthy people from your company died under similar circumstances within six months of each other and the police department was asked to carry out an investigation. We're looking into everything. We want to make sure there were no problems at work or threats to deal with."

"But what does that matter?" Phil shook his head. "They both died during surgery by the same doctor. Maybe that's where you should be asking questions and looking into work habits."

"Fair enough and we plan to do that once we finish here. Did Mr.

Burdette ever have a problem with the finances? Any discrepancies that you were aware of or concerned about?"

Phil sighed as he looked at his desk. "We were having a few problems with balancing the books. The problem was pointed out to me and we immediately called him in for questioning as well as an action plan for remediation."

"And how was that progressing?" Alex asked.

Phil looked at him as if he forgot Alex was in the room. "We hadn't gotten too far into things before Frank passed away."

"And Connie? Didn't she work with Frank, in the same department?"

"Yes, she was his secretary, if you can use that term anymore."

"Would it be safe to say she would know if any money went missing?"

"Not necessarily," Phil said shrugging his shoulders. "She certainly completed any paperwork he needed but I'm not sure how much she was aware of numbers."

Jake leaned forward and asked his next question with a grin. "Were they close? Outside of work, did they see each other?"

Phil immediately shrugged. "How the hell would I know or even care for that matter? There were some problems with the books but I don't see how that matters since their death was related to botched surgery. Like I said, you should go after the doctor."

Jake sat back and smiled. "I assure you, sir, we are in discussion with the doctor and plan to follow up on every angle. I have one more question about MemorHold."

"What?" Phil sighed as he looked at his watch once again. "Make it quick because I have to go."

"Your company? Do you have silent partners? Investors?"

"Of course we do. We even have a board of directors and everyone else that makes the life of a corporate CEO a nightmare. As a result, there's an internal auditor for the books. Now if you don't mind leaving, I do have a meeting I have to be in." Phil quickly leaned forward and stabbed a button on his phone to summon his administrative assistant to come in and retrieve the men.

Her smile lit the room when she saw Jake and she was eager to escort the men to the front desk. "I believe you were going to leave your name and number for me," she said from hooded eyes. "I've written my information down for you." She handed Jake a small slip of perfumed paper as he casually pulled up a pant leg and sat on the corner of her desk. He smiled as he looked at it and placed it in inside his jacket pocket.

"Thank you."

She handed him another slip of perfumed paper along with a pen. Jake spent a moment writing down his name and number and handed it back to her. She smiled and place it inside a tiny purse.

Flashing her a winning smile, he stood and the two men left the office.

As they walked toward the car, Alex shook his head and stared at him. "Really, dude? Do you just keep collecting names and numbers wherever you go?"

Jake laughed. "She's not my type, but it never hurts to have an inside person if you need sensitive information."

"That's even worse. You're going to string her along?"

"No, I'll just keep the number in case I need to call. I didn't ask her out."

"Not yet, anyway." Alex grabbed the passenger door and slipped inside as Jake got behind the wheel. Jake shot him a look as he fired up the engine knowing Alex would be surprised if he could read his mind at the moment.

# CHAPTER 41

Elizabeth pulled into the parking deck of the hospital and parked the car. It was early morning and she was scheduled for surgery for the first time in ten days. She felt more relaxed than she had in awhile and realized there was a small spark of joy and perhaps hope now that she had a theory about the deaths of her patients.

She went into the locker room and changed into scrubs. She locked her clothes away as well as her purse and keys. Donning a cover, she made her way into the pre-op area where she took the time to review the records of her surgical patient. Mr. Jackson was a middle-aged man who had an abdominal tumor which had to be removed. He had experienced pain in his abdomen and was sent for a CT scan which revealed the mass. The recommendation had been for immediate removal and biopsy. Elizabeth reviewed his meds carefully, making sure he was not taking anything that might thin his blood, specifically asking about garlic and other supplements.

"Where is he?" Elizabeth asked the nurse at the pre-op desk.

"Your patient is in cubicle number two," the nurse said as she held up two manicured fingers. A clear cut sign she didn't assist in any surgery or provide direct care as she would have had to lop those nails off in a nano-second.

"Thanks," Elizabeth said as she put down his paper chart and made her way to the cubicle.

"Mr. Jackson, how are you today?" He was lying on a gurney layered with green fabric. His body was barely covered by a hospital gown and he was wearing a surgical hairnet over his head.

"I'm about as good as I could hope for," he said with a shrug. "You know, I'd rather be anywhere except here. Who knows what you're gonna find."

"I'm sorry you feel that way," she said. "I know it's unpleasant to have to be here and who knows why this mass started growing, but you'll be much better off when it's out. Then we can worry about what to do with it."

"Whatever," he said as he turned his face away.

"Mr. Jackson, please look at me," Elizabeth said kindly. When he finally turned his head, she said, "I swear I will do my absolute best to make sure you have a great experience in this OR. I have to ask you once again and you have to be absolutely honest with me. Are you taking any blood thinners or any supplements that would act like a blood thinner?"

She watched as he shook his head.

"Great, have you ever had a supplement by the name of Memor-Hold or anything similar that you know of?"

Once again, he shook his head more vigorously.

"And no mysterious bruises, bumps, fevers or episodes of severe fatigue."

"No, no and no," he said as he looked at her and frowned at the same time. "Look, Doc, I don't mean to whine but can we just get it over with? Sitting around here is making me so anxious I'm gonna jump off the gurney."

Elizabeth reached out and patted his arm. "Yes, I'm going to tell them to get moving. You hang on, okay? I'll talk to you again in recovery."

"If I'm lucky," he said as he squeezed her hand back.

Elizabeth walked out, wrote a note on the chart and handed it back to the pre-op nurse. "Okay, tell the team to move him into the OR while I go scrub."

# CHAPTER 42

"So what's next?" Alex asked as Jake drove. Jake hadn't talked much since they left MemorHold the day before which was very unusual for him. "Hello, earth to Jake? What's eating you? You've never been this quiet."

Jake turned to look at his partner. "I'm just trying to figure this out. I feel like we're missing something." Jake was thinking about how defensive he felt when Phil Harry started maligning Elizabeth Brooks. He didn't believe she was involved, or had any reason to hurt those employees, and his intuition was usually spot on. But he usually wasn't bothered by feeling over protective either. "What did you think of Harry?"

"Other than he's a complete arrogant ass?" Alex asked.

"Yea, I think that part was pretty obvious. His employees, the little people, are clearly beneath him."

"I hate people who think they're better than others."

"I hear ya, pal. So, I want to ask you once again about Dr. Brooks."

"What about her?" Alex turned to Jake, curiosity written over his face.

"I want to make sure she's clean. You checked her bank accounts and her profile, right? You didn't see any evidence of her recently receiving extra money, or large deposits or having anything that would be considered a profit or a bribe?"

"I found nothing," Alex said, shaking his head. "She has the same profile as any new doctor. Loan obligations for her office, condo, and car. She works long hours, doesn't have anything to brag about such as expensive art, a large estate, fancy jewelry or cars. No obligations," Alex said as he emphasized the next words, "such as husbands, past or present."

Jake tightened his hands on the steering wheel as he listened to Alex's report. "So, to be sure, there would be no secondary gain or reason for her to risk her career, her reputation or a criminal offense by purposely screwing up surgery and killing patients."

"Sounds kind of ridiculous hearing it out loud," Alex said as he looked out the window.

"I agree, but I want to be sure we're not thinking in that direction before we proceed," Jake said. "I think we need to talk to Connie's friend, the one who visited her husband. She may have more knowledge of what's going on at MemorHold. Hell, she may know of more cases that we haven't gotten wind of."

"I'll get the number and reach out tomorrow. We can go tomorrow afternoon if she's free," Alex said.

"I can't go tomorrow. I have a meeting with the Captain. Probably going to chew me out again."

Alex laughed as he turned to Jake. "Are you kidding me? If anyone is made of teflon in this department, it's you."

Jake remained quiet. "Listen, if you can get hold of her, you go and do the interview. We need to start moving on this. Something's going to break soon. I can feel it in my bones."

Alex continued to look out the window and laugh.

# CHAPTER 43

Elizabeth pulled off her gloves and untied her surgical mask. Turning around, she threw her surgical gown into the proper receptacle. Elizabeth was pleased the surgery had gone well. Reviewing her post-op orders, she was hopeful all would continue to go well with her patient. She left instructions to monitor his blood pressure, oxygen level, mental status, and lab to ensure he didn't have any early signs of bleeding. After reviewing the orders, she went into his electronic medical record and wrote her surgical procedure note, including technique and exact details of suture, instruments and post-op dressing.

As she was locking her documentation, she was called by one of the recovery nurses to see her patient. Feeling a knot in her stomach, she went into recovery before changing. She walked up to the nursing station and asked for the specific nurse who had called her.

"Melissa, is everything okay?" Elizabeth realized her heart rate was faster than usual and she felt a bit breathless.

Melissa looked up from the chart she was working on. "Hi, Dr. Brooks. Yes, everything's fine, but Mr. Jackson woke up and he's insisting on seeing you immediately."

"Okay, I'll speak with him. Do you have any idea what his concern is?"

Melissa shook her head. "No, he seems fine. Vitals are stable, he got his pain meds, anesthesia has worn off and his dressing was checked."

Elizabeth nodded. "Thank you. I'll go see him now." He was lying in his bed, his eyes closed. His face appeared relaxed and his breathing was even.

"Mr. Jackson, it's Dr Brooks. You wanted to see me?" Elizabeth spoke softly as the recovery room was currently hushed due to the condition of most of the patients.

Mr. Jackson's eyelids fluttered as he turned his face toward Elizabeth. She watched him as he turned. He appeared a bit lethargic from the medication, but he was responsive and smiled. He reached out and took her hand. With a hoarse whisper, he said, "Dr. Brooks."

Leaning closer to him, she said, "Yes, I'm here. Are you okay?"

He slowly nodded his head. "Maybe it's the medicine, but I'm feeling really well."

"I'm happy to hear that," Elizabeth said. "When the nurse said you wanted to see me, I was concerned you were having pain or another problem."

He shook his head. "No, I wanted to tell you. I felt I had to tell you immediately. I feel well and I had a vision while I was under. He told me I was fine and would heal quickly." Mr. Jackson looked up at Elizabeth as tears filled his eyes.

Elizabeth squeezed his hand. "What's wrong? I don't understand."

"I just want to thank you. You saved my life and I'll spend many happy years with my family."

Elizabeth swallowed as she held his hand. "Mr. Jackson, that would be a wonderful outcome, but I do want to remind you we have to wait for the official biopsy to come back from the pathologist. Once we have that, we can decide what we're going to do next."

Mr. Jackson nodded as he cried. "It's benign. I am so blessed, it's benign." He looked up at Elizabeth. "He told me it's benign and to thank you for saving my life. He said there was a moment when a surgeon with less steady hands could have cut the wrong thing, but you're a superstar and saved my life. I'm going to tell everyone when I get out of the hospital."

Elizabeth felt her stomach knot again. There had been a small moment during surgery when his anatomy had become difficult to navigate, but she was able to properly identify the right vessel and complete surgery without problems. But Mr. Jackson wouldn't have known that.

Smiling, Elizabeth said, "You're fine. Sometimes anesthesia can make you feel very emotional. I promise we'll talk again later. You should try to get some sleep and rest. The more you rest, the faster you'll heal and get the heck out of the hospital." Silently, she prayed that his biopsy returned with a benign diagnosis.

"I will, Doctor. Now that I know I'll be with my family for a long time." He started to chuckle while he spoke. "Oh, yeah, one more thing."

"What's that?" Elizabeth said.

"Frank said to say, Hi."

Elizabeth froze when she heard what he said. "Say that again?"

"The vision, was a man. He said his name was Frank and he spoke to me during the surgery. He kept me calm and he assured me the biopsy would be normal and to tell you, he said, Hi."

Swallowing hard, Elizabeth felt like she could barely breathe. She was speechless for a few seconds as her mind raced.

"Hey Doc, you okay?"

Elizabeth nodded as she realized her patient was now asking after her welfare. "Yes, I'm fine. Thank you for telling me this. I'm sure you're going to heal very quickly." She straightened his blanket. "Now, you rest and I'll see you again, very soon."

Mr. Jackson nodded. "You've got it, Doc."

Elizabeth smiled, turned on her heel and walked away.

# CHAPTER 44

Jake parked the car and removed his seat belt. "What was the friend's name again?"

"Deborah Turner," Alex said as he opened his door. "I started collecting information the minute we left Connie Arturo's house. There's nothing exciting, no credit card issues, no warrants, no large bank accounts anywhere."

"But she is an employee of MemorHold?"

"As far as I can tell, she's still an active employee of MemorHold," Alex said as he got out and looked at Jake over the top of the car.

"Then you're going to see her. Ask her about the free pills. See if she can tell you anything suspicious about the company. Find out who her manager is. Someone will talk."

The two men walked into the police station. "What will you be doing while I'm investigating?"

"I'm going to follow up on a couple of leads, and I have to talk to the chief," Jake said. "There's something fishy about that company and I'm going to find out what it is. I want more angles on this. The employees, the product, the silent partners, the CEO. We're missing something and damn it all, I'm going to find out what it is."

"Because you don't want to ruin your record or because you have another interest?" Alex said as they walked into the squad room and headed over to their desks.

Jake gestured to Alex and walked to his desk. "I have a few contacts and inside informants that I want to reach out to, but I can't do it while we're together. No offense, but I've cultivated their trust over many years and I can't risk that now. So you go to Deborah Turner and see what you can get. I'm calling in a few favors and then we'll share our info."

"Aye, aye." Alex frowned as he gave Jake a mock salute. He shook his head as he mumbled about taking orders from Jake. They hadn't worked together long and Jake was one of his more difficult partners, but Jake did have a stellar record and having that relationship as part of his career path certainly wouldn't hurt, as long as he could stand it.

# CHAPTER 45

Elizabeth walked into the café, grabbed a bite and sat down in a corner of the physician's lounge. Within five minutes, Caitlyn sauntered into the area. "Hey, can a nurse join you in here or will I be vaporized if I enter without invitation?"

Elizabeth looked up. "Consider yourself invited."

"Gee thanks, don't sound so excited," Caitlyn said as she pulled out a chair and sat next to Elizabeth.

"Sorry, I just got out of surgery."

"Everything okay?" Caitlyn looked at her with wide eyes, hoping she wouldn't hear about another unexpected complication.

Pausing for a moment, Elizabeth finally answered. "Yeah, he's fine. The surgery went well, but I'm waiting for the biopsy to come back. From the size of the growth I'm a little worried."

"But?" Caitlyn stared at her friend as she sipped a cup of soup.

"But what?"

"There's a big but in there. I can tell from your face, so keep going."

Elizabeth shrugged as she frowned. "He was acting a bit strange in post-op. He said he had a vision and he knows the tumor is benign and he thanked me." Elizabeth shook her head. "I don't know when the hell things got so strange in my career, but it's a lot different than it was in medical school."

Caitlyn laughed. "There's a reason for everything. You just don't know what it is, yet."

"Let's hope that's true." Elizabeth put her empty cup on the table.

"Well, I have something which may give you a start."

"Really? Like what?"

"The information you asked me about?"

"Yes?" Elizabeth held her breath.

"I went through most of the record and I didn't find much, but then I looked at what the patient had written by hand on a medication list when he came to the hospital. Medical records scanned the paper into the chart to be complete."

"And?" Elizabeth was getting impatient.

Caitlyn stopped talking as another doctor paused near the entrance of the physician's lounge. After a moment, she turned to Elizabeth and said, "It's a beautiful day outside. I can't wait to get off shift."

Elizabeth felt herself tense as they waited for the lounge to clear. When it did, she turned to Caitlyn.

"Quick, what did you find?"

"Apparently, the patient listed the MemorHold supplements on the paper when he filled out the paperwork by hand, but for some reason it never made the medication list in the computer. I don't know who filled out the chart, but someone's head is going to roll. That's for sure. I don't even know if Pruitt or Risk Management has figured it out yet."

Elizabeth turned her chair toward her friend and grabbed her arm. "Wait, so you're telling me that the patient who died during surgery with Dr. Pruitt was also taking MemorHold, but it was missed because someone didn't enter it on the medical record?"

Caitlyn nodded and pointed to her nose. "Bingo. On the other hand, MemorHold is not on a watch list at this point."

"But that's it," Elizabeth said. "I think we have enough to assume it's MemorHold. No one regulates it because it's a supplement." Elizabeth was pensive for a moment. "I think it's time for me to go to the Safety Reporting Portal."

"Well, just cover your bases. I can't give you any info because I shouldn't have been in that chart at this point, but I can guarantee someone will want to know this information."

"That's the point. From this moment on, we screen everyone with pending surgery as to whether they've taken the med."

"Obviously, you can do whatever you wish for your patients. I don't know what the hospital protocol is for a situation like this, but you should find out before you do anything publicly."

"You know I will," Elizabeth said, excitement and hope creeping into her voice. "Think of the people we can save if we make this information public."

"Think of the liability you'll face if you're wrong. Let the professionals do their job and move along."

"Thank you, thank you so much," Elizabeth said as she hugged her friend.

Caitlyn pushed her away. "I'm serious, whatever you do, make sure you keep my name out of it." She stood, picked up her soup cup and strode out of the lounge.

# CHAPTER 46

Finishing at the hospital, Elizabeth visited Mr. Jackson before she left. He was doing well, his pain had decreased and he was excited about going home as soon as possible. He held fast to his vision that his tumor was benign and he would be good as new.

Elizabeth drove to the office and entered through her private back door. She placed her purse and keys in her bottom desk drawer and situated herself in her chair. Quickly scanning her messages, she prioritized them into call back piles according to their content. She then reviewed the lab on her desk, initialed everything she read and made a separate pile of normal lab results. Her staff would be able to call those patients and let them know of the outcome. She kept all abnormal results for herself.

Just as she finished, Heather knocked on the door and let herself in. "Hey, I thought I heard you."

"Here I am," Elizabeth said, smiling at Heather.

Looking at the desk, she said, "I'm glad you found the lab and messages. I didn't let anyone touch anything until you reviewed it all."

"Thanks, I appreciate it," Elizabeth said. "It's very important I review everything now." Elizabeth handed her the pile of normal lab results. "These can be called back today. Please let the patients know they were normal. I put a note on each one as to when they need to come back for another test."

"Okay, great," Heather said as she turned away.

"No wait," Elizabeth said. "Did you find out anything about MemorHold for our patients?"

"Yes, I left you a list." Heather walked over and shuffled through the papers on the side of the desk. She pulled out a yellow lined sheet of paper and handed it to Elizabeth. "I went through as many charts as I could yesterday afternoon. I can tell you that the two patients who died after surgery this year were both taking the supplement. There are a few others who have it listed on their med list."

"Have you had time to call any of them?"

"Not yet, but I will. What do you want me to ask? Are you alive?"

"No, tell them we want to check on them. If they have an appointment due, make it sound like we're giving them an appointment reminder. Then mention they should let us know if they have any extra bruising or problems so we can make sure we get lab work when they come to the office." Elizabeth nodded at Heather. "You know how to do it."

"Yeah, I'll think of something," Heather said with a grin.

"Keep checking charts and make a list of which patients are taking it. It's so important." Elizabeth smiled as she looked up at Heather.

"I got it," Heather said.

"And if anyone says they're not feeling well, you tell them to stop taking that supplement immediately. By the way, did you get hold of Lucky?"

"I called him but he didn't answer the phone."

"Please keep trying. Maybe he's out for the night?"

Heather laughed as she turned toward the door. "Where? Oh sure, he had tickets for Broadway in Manhattan tonight."

Elizabeth cleared her throat and shot Heather a nasty look.

"Okay, okay. Sorry, Boss. Let me start working on it and then I can bring you another pile to review."

"Thank you," Elizabeth said with a frown as she watched Heather go. The minute the door closed, Elizabeth booted up her computer and navigated to the FDA Safety Reporting Portal. She was excited as she was convinced the MemorHold supplement was the cause of a lot of problems, many of them not even realized. She logged in and entered her claim. She typed her information, being as anonymous as she was allowed. She put in as much information as she could and finally exited the program. Her claim would be reviewed and dependent on the level of concern, it could be expedited. She was hoping that MemorHold would be receiving a visit from the FDA soon. At least the process was started and if she was wrong, then so be it. But if she was right, and the medicine was capable of causing hemorrhage, weak vessels and death, thousands of lives would be saved. Elizabeth wasn't sure exactly what the interaction was, but if they could prove a causal relationship then that was enough.

Once she was finished for the day, Elizabeth packed her things and slipped out her private door. She locked up and drove home, tired and hungry. After picking up her mail, she went inside and threw her things on the counter. She kicked off her shoes and checked for messages. Seeing none, she quickly sorted through her mail.

Elizabeth opened the refrigerator and pulled out fresh vegetables to make a salad sprinkled with grilled chicken. Picking up a bottle of water, she sat down and enjoyed her salad while watching the news.

Once she was done, she walked her dishes to the sink and was about to go into the bedroom when her cell phone rang. Checking the caller ID she noticed it was her father and picked up.

"Hey, Dad."

"Hey, yourself. How was your day?"

"It was interesting. I think I'm making progress with that little problem I had."

"Oh, really? What happened?"

"Well, based on our conversation this weekend, I had Heather start looking into the charts of all my patients. I found a few people on the supplement, MemorHold. The two people who died after surgery were on it as well. Then, I found out there was another death in the Surgical ICU, but it wasn't one of my patients. It was a patient of pissant Pruitt."

"You're kidding me?"

"No, not at all. Anyway, I got someone to look into the chart for me."

"Hey, what did we say about being careful."

"I was and I know I shouldn't have but I needed to know. The supplement wasn't on his med list, but there was a piece of paper scanned into the chart that listed the supplement."

"What's the name of this pill again?"

"MemorHold. It's made by a company of the same name and it supposedly keeps your mind sharp and helps prevent memory loss."

"Maybe I should get some of that stuff," Parker said.

"Dad, stop."

"Okay, relax. I was just teasing."

"Can you do me a favor?"

"What?"

"Can you call John Donovan and ask him if he would know if any of the people he was having trouble with at the funeral home were taking that supplement. Or if anyone specifically had weak vessels or a burst vessel? I know it's a lot but maybe there's something he can piece together."

"I'll call him," Parker said. "I'm not sure how much information he gets when he picks up a body, but there's no harm in asking."

"Great, thank you, Dad. Did you get the records I mailed yet?"

"Not yet, maybe tomorrow. Is there a nutritionist you can check with at the hospital? She may be up to date on supplements and complications."

"That's a great idea, Dad."

"So, when are you coming back to the shore?"

Elizabeth laughed as she said, "Dad, I was just there a couple of days ago."

"I know, but having you here reminded us how much we miss you. Goldy has been depressed since the moment you left. She won't eat or play. She keeps going to the front door and whining. When I ask her what's up, she looks at the front door and barks. She's pining after you so you may as well come back and calm her down."

"She's a great dog. Maybe I'll take a ride down this weekend. There's been some developments and I want to make sure I have time to follow up with them." Elizabeth paused for a moment. "It's important, Dad. It may help my case at the hospital and with the lawsuit."

"I get it, Lizzie. I get it. You know, I was thinking of visiting North Jersey, so maybe the three of us will take a little ride up this weekend. Your mother and I haven't been to New Wales in a long while. We'll get a hotel, but we'd have to find one that accepts pets."

"Oh no, I have a beautiful guest room. You can stay here."

"That's great. Goldy will be thrilled. Maybe we can have some fun this weekend. And then, where do you want to go for Sunday dinner? You don't have to cook. We could go out to a restaurant."

"But then, Goldy can't go."

"We'll order in then, but don't cook. It would be better if you spent time with Goldy."

Laughing she said, "Okay, call me in the morning, just in case something changes. It will be great to see you."

"You've got it, Lizzie. It's a date. Your mother and I would love to see your place."

"Sounds great. I'm looking forward to it as well."

"Sleep tight. Lock all your doors and windows. Be safe."

"I will, Dad. Any reason why you're particularly concerned?"

"No, just a Dad thing. Listen, I don't know exactly what you're getting into up there, but let the professionals handle the problem. I don't want you getting yourself into trouble."

"I will. Don't worry."

"Famous last words," Parker said as he cleared his throat. Elizabeth could hear Goldy barking in the background as if she was agreeing with him.

"Gotta go, love you."

"Love you too, Lizzie. See you soon."

Elizabeth clicked off the call, turned off the lights and walked into the bedroom. She stripped off her clothes, and took a hot shower to release some of the tension of the day. After toweling off, she dressed in a silky night dress and snuggled into bed. She was tired, but felt hopeful for the first time in a long while. If the FDA agreed with her claim, she would be exonerated.

She felt sleepy as she snuggled into the pillows and slowly relaxed enough to drift off to sleep.

The dream started out peacefully.

*She walked along a path in the woods. She wasn't sure if it was the same path she'd seen before, but something was different. The trees were swaying in the wind and the sky was dark as if a storm was brewing. She could smell the damp earth as big drops of rain hit the area. Walking forward, she headed for the trees and saw a small shed in the woods. Elizabeth was always told not to stand under a tree during a storm, but she was afraid to stand in the open. Reaching forward, she opened the door to the shed and stepped inside....*

Elizabeth's cell phone rang and startled her from sleep. She pulled the phone off the side table and pushed the green button. Mumbling, she spoke into the phone. "Lo?"

"Dr. Brooks?" A strong female voice.

"Yes, can I help you?" Elizabeth asked, beginning to wake.

"This is Becky from the Surgical ICU."

Elizabeth felt her stomach clench as she sat up.

"Yes?"

"Sorry to wake you up. I'm calling about Mr. Jackson."

"Is everything okay?" Elizabeth asked, panic spreading through her.

"Yes, Doctor, it's just that he's complaining of pain."

"I left prn orders on the chart. Did you medicate him?"

"That's just it. You gave us an opioid order. Mr. Jackson says he feels so good, he only wants acetaminophen, but we don't have an order for that. Can I have an order?"

Elizabeth took a deep breath to calm herself. She tucked a strand of hair behind her ear. "Of course." She rattled off the recommended dose and frequency and had the nurse read the verbal order back to her.

"Thank you, Doctor," Becky said as she hung up the phone.

Elizabeth put the phone on the charger and fell back against the pillows. She was sure she wouldn't be able to sleep now, her heart was pounding and her breathing was heavy. When the nurse identified herself, Elizabeth was expecting her to say that Mr. Jackson had a severe complication. As much as she was frightened of Mr. Jackson's dream, she hoped he would be right about his health. She knew he had a high chance of being diagnosed with cancer, so a benign biopsy would be welcomed. Even if it was benign, it didn't mean that Frank had anything to do with it.

The dreams with Frank were evolving but she hadn't told anyone about the content of the dreams. Elizabeth sat up, grabbed her knees and rocked herself. It was time to face the fear she had all along. The fear her parents had when she was young. She had been to many doctors. They checked to make sure she wasn't imagining things or attention seeking. She was checked for tumors, seizures and any other abnormalities. Trying their best to be good parents, and providing her with all the medical attention she needed, Parker and C.J. had her examined by an internist, neurologist, psychiatrist, social worker and sleep medicine specialist. She was screened for anxiety, panic, depression, PTSD, seizures, and sleep apnea. As a result she was prescribed medication, cognitive behavioral therapy, counseling and exercise to induce fatigue.

When she was young, Elizabeth took a small amount of medication, then held most of it between her gum and cheek until she could spit it out. She endured the counseling, and behavioral therapy, but she enjoyed the exercise. Running allowed her to let her thoughts simply float.

The dreams didn't go away, but Elizabeth stopped talking about them. When she was questioned, she denied having them although she admitted she didn't always sleep well.

The dreams started after Elizabeth was in a horrible accident. She was off from school and spent the day with her mother. They enjoyed a great day together, shopping, eating and stopping at the playground. On their way home, Elizabeth skipped ahead on the sidewalk. C.J. saw the drunk driver coming toward them. His car swerved and wandered all over the road. Too late, she realized Elizabeth was directly in the path of the car and ran toward her. Unfortunately, she didn't make it in time. The car jumped the curb and hit Elizabeth before C.J. could reach her. Her screams were heard by many when she saw her daughter's body sprawled on the sidewalk, a pool of blood surrounding her head.

Elizabeth was Medevaced to the nearest trauma hospital. She was immediately treated and worked up. Her injuries needed a lot of care and she was finally discharged from the hospital exactly one month after she was admitted. Her body had healed by the time the dreams began. After assuming the dreams were a normal response to her trauma, the doctors tried counseling and medications. When nothing helped, they wondered if Elizabeth was seeking attention. It was clear that her dreams were stressful for all. Eventually, Elizabeth stopped talking about them but they surfaced again in high school. So, the doctors and counseling started all over again until Elizabeth stopped sharing.

The dreams frightened Elizabeth and she told her parents and doctors that she dreamt of dead people, but after many hours of questions and treatments, Elizabeth realized it was better to keep them to herself. The treatments didn't help and the dreams didn't always go away.

The one aspect they never discussed and didn't want to face was whether the dreams could actually represent paranormal activity. Elizabeth thought about it a lot when she was a child but never talked about it for fear they would lock her up. People talked to her in her dreams. She tried to test her theory in medical school but could never prove she was experiencing anything more than exaggerated REM sleep and insomnia. The dreams came and went depending on the level of stress she was under.

Frank was harder to ignore. Over the last several months, she'd gone through all the same emotions, but chalked her dreams up to the stress she endured from the guilt of losing a patient. Then she'd lost two. She wasn't surprised and waited for the full fledged panic disorder to start. Returning to her meditation and stress exercises, she had been able to hold her own, but having Mr. Jackson talk about Frank threw her for a loop. It scared her to think that Frank could really be reaching out to her, not only through her dreams but the dreams of others.

She felt frightened when she saw him, felt him, heard him, but he never threatened her. Elizabeth fell back to the pillows and buried herself within her comforter. After counting to one hundred she began to feel sleepy.

*SHE LOOKED up and realized she was standing at the door of the shed. It was dark inside, but it was stormy outside and she was frightened. "C'mon in, I promise I won't bite."*

*Startled, Elizabeth realized she was now in the middle of the shed. Frank was standing near her, studying her face.*

*"It's time to stop being nervous. I need you to have complete focus here."*

*Elizabeth looked at the man before her. He seemed completely real, completely whole, but how?*

*"I need you to understand, you're heading in the right direction, but it's not without danger. Things have now been set in motion. You have to keep going but you have to be careful."*

*"How are you talking to me if I'm dreaming?" Elizabeth heard the words in her head but didn't feel her mouth move. How odd.*

*"I don't have enough time to explain, Liz."*

*Elizabeth felt herself stiffen in her dream.*

*"It's okay, I can call you Dr. Brooks if it makes you feel more comfortable. But since I'm dead and you're able to hear me, I think we can be on more comfortable terms. Listen closely, I don't have a lot of time to visit with you, it exhausts me. I tried to prove this is real when I sent the message through Roy Jackson. He's so happy he's going to live a long happy life."*

*"But how did you...?"*

*"No time, Liz." Frank weakened. "Your friend Jake visited with Phil Harry. Things are in motion. You must be careful. Be very careful."*

ELIZABETH SAT UPRIGHT IN BED. She began to shake and cry. Jolts of adrenaline shot through her body. She threw her legs over the side of the bed and held onto the table. Walking to the bathroom, she turned on the light and drank a glass of water. She took a cold wash cloth and wiped her face. Just a dream. It was just a dream. Or was it?

Elizabeth walked back to the bed and sat down. She took several deep breaths and picked up her phone. She rarely liked to waste time surfing the net, but it served as a great distraction when needed.

Elizabeth activated her phone and checked out several social media apps. She scrolled through and saw plenty of posts about flowers, dogs and prayer requests. She was tempted to research paranormal activity through dreams but didn't want to spend time reading unsubstantiated claims. After fifteen minutes, she felt more relaxed and actually felt drained. A few minutes after that, she was curled up and sound asleep for the third time that night.

# CHAPTER 47

Elizabeth woke to sunlight streaming through her windows. The pounding in her head gave notice of her headache. She knew she had a dream last night. As she concentrated, she was able to remember the details and completely focus. She had been visited by Frank. Had he visited or did she dream about him? The only thing Elizabeth knew was he warned her about danger. He said things were set in motion and she was now in danger.

Jumping out of bed, she quickly showered and dressed for work. She wasn't frightened, but felt nervous and confused. Was Frank real or was he a dream? It was important. If he was real, she was in real danger. If he was a dream, she could still be in danger. But from what? It was one thing to avoid someone or a particular place but it was very difficult when you didn't know what to watch out for.

Elizabeth drove to the hospital and made her post-op rounds. Roy Jackson was doing well and was able to move to a regular room. Elizabeth was thrilled for him and had the distinct pleasure of letting him know that his biopsy did indeed return as a benign growth. Once Roy was healed, he could return to a full healthy life.

Next, she went to medical records and completed her notes. She wanted to be completely clear and exact when she had to sit in front of her peers and defend her surgical record. She had reviewed the records over and over and her technique was flawless. If she could prove Memorhold had been the reason her patient suffered unexpected complications, she could exonerate her record.

Walking back to the café, Elizabeth ran into Caitlyn in the hall.

"Hi, how are things going?" Elizabeth asked.

"Fine for me, how about by you?"

"Well, things are well," Elizabeth said as she nodded her head.

Caitlyn pulled her aside. "You're lying. You look like crap. Have you slept at all in the last month?"

"I've slept in the last month, just not last night." Elizabeth entered the café and walked over to the coffee bar. She turned to Caitlyn and lowered her voice. "I'm sorry I asked you to look into that chart. It was so important for me to make that connection but I didn't want you to feel uncomfortable. I didn't realize you were angry until yesterday."

Caitlyn looked down at her cup. "I'm sorry I was crabby. I was able to get into the chart because I was part of the surgical team. There's so much tension around here, I don't want to get in the middle of it."

Elizabeth put her arm around Caitlyn's shoulders. "I'm sorry. If I ever ask you to do anything stupid again, just tell me and walk away."

Caitlyn looked at her watch. "By my count, that should be tomorrow."

"Shut up," Elizabeth said as she frowned at her friend. "I'm trying to be contrite here."

Caitlyn laughed until she saw Dr. Pruitt walk into the café. She turned and made a hasty retreat to the far side of the room.

Elizabeth walked over to a table in the physician's lounge and sat down, purposely avoiding Caitlyn so she wouldn't feel uncomfortable. After three minutes or so, Dr. Pruitt walked into the physician's lounge and spied her in the corner, sipping coffee. He sat at a table in the middle of the lounge and set his coffee down with a bang. Elizabeth looked up but didn't take the bait when he looked toward her. She continued to scroll through her phone.

Several quiet minutes went by. "Dr. Brooks?"

Elizabeth's head snapped up. "Yes, Dr. Pruitt?"

"You're looking awfully relaxed," his voice boomed.

"Is there something wrong with that?" She asked in a sweet voice.

"You do understand you'll be sitting in front of the department next week as they consider suspending your privileges?"

"I understand that's your goal," Elizabeth answered.

"I only want what's right for the patients."

"I see," she said. "Will they be considering your surgical skill as well?"

"Excuse me?" His face turned bright red.

"Oh, I'm sorry. I thought I overheard someone say your last patient had unfortunately died in the surgical ICU. Perhaps I misunderstood."

His face turned completely red as she pointed out his gaffe. "That is a completely different matter."

"Really? I don't think it is and I plan to point it out when I do speak in front of the department and administration next week."

Pruitt stood up abruptly. "What does that mean?"

Elizabeth resisted the urge to smile. "To be honest, I've been looking back at my patient's charts and their surgical reports. I've read them over and over. I believe I've found the problem and I plan to present it as soon as possible for the safety of the hospital and community as a whole."

"What in the hell are you talking about?" Pruitt yelled.

Elizabeth got up and walked over to Pruitt although he was taller than her by a good ten inches. "The problem is a new supplement called MemorHold."

Pruitt looked incredulous for ten seconds. "What?"

"MemorHold. It's new in the community and every patient who died was taking that supplement." When Elizabeth saw his face, she stuttered a little. "Well, I don't know about your patient, but at least mine were taking it. It hasn't been well studied because it's a supplement but hopefully I was able to do something about that."

Pruitt turned purple as he stared at her. "What did you do?"

Excitement took over as Elizabeth was proud of her sleuthing skills. "I put a claim into the FDA Safety Portal. I'm hoping Memor-

Hold gets a call any day now from the FDA. If they find enough of a concern, they'll have the media put out a notification to pull all the MemorHold they can find.

Pruitt was eerily quiet when he spoke. "Are you trying to tell me that you're blaming the deaths of your patients on a common supplement that they may or may not have been taking? Are you trying to offload your responsibility as a surgeon and clinician onto a little pill?"

Nodding, Elizabeth stepped back. A small niggle of doubt in her mind. "Yes, I think the supplement was responsible for a change in their response to surgery or anesthesia and I'm pushing to have it studied before a hundred more people die. I think it affects the vascular system."

"That is the most ridiculous thing I've ever heard."

"Both of my deceased patients had a complication which was nowhere near my surgical field and did not show up on any of the scans performed before surgery. Whether you want to believe it or not, Dr. Pruitt, there are times people die of complications that have nothing to do with the surgeon or your quality data. I find it very interesting you're so willing to boot me off the staff but I guess you hold yourself above everyone else. Well, we'll see about that." Elizabeth stood tall as she defended herself. "Instead of worrying about me, I'd suggest you look through your own patient's chart. You may want to hear more about my research."

She walked around Pruitt as he stood there looking like he was about to blow. Once she cleared the doorway of the physician's lounge, she quickly scooted into the ladies room across the hall and locked herself into the large stall. Bracing herself against the wall, she took deep breaths as her heart raced and her dizziness threatened to envelope her.

"Elizabeth? Elizabeth are you in here?" Caitlyn had followed her into the ladies room.

After a few seconds of silence, the stall door clicked as Elizabeth slowly opened the door. "Yes, I'm in here."

"Are you alright?"

"I'm a little shaky," Elizabeth said with a small smile. "Did you hear us?"

Eyebrows raised, Caitlyn said, "I think everyone in the whole damn building heard you. I don't know why, but this man is after your head."

"I'm tired of it. As a matter of fact, he's going to be slapped with a lawsuit for harassment if he keeps it up."

"Well, it certainly didn't sound as if you were whimpering when he threatened you."

Elizabeth suddenly started to laugh. "As a matter of fact, I thought he was going to rupture his own vessel due to apoplexy." She continued to laugh, almost hysterically. "He deserved it, that asshat is over the top." Elizabeth's shoulders continued to shake, although Caitlyn realized her friend was now crying as the emotions poured out. She walked over and hugged her as she sobbed.

"Hey, you've fought months of emotions and you have to pick my lunch hour to release it all?"

Elizabeth chuckled as she clung to her friend. Caitlyn reached over and wet a paper towel and wiped Elizabeth's face. "Listen, things are getting more intense as that blowhard gets closer to challenging your privileges here. Let's face it, things may get a little more intense until everything is done, but you really need to get some rest and compose yourself. I know you don't want to take a leave but it would be a good idea to make sure your schedule stays light until this is over."

Nodding, Elizabeth hugged her friend once more and sighed.

"You look exhausted. Why don't you cancel the rest of your day and go home and sleep. Take a pill if you have to, but you need to get some rest."

"You're right. I'm so tired."

"Then get your stuff together and get the heck out of here."

# CHAPTER 48

It was strange arriving home in the middle of the day. Elizabeth felt off but admitted she was too tired to fight. She put her bag and keys down, changed into yoga pants and a T-shirt, turned off her bedroom light and plopped onto the bed. Her plan was to simply be quiet and relax, but she fell asleep within a few minutes. Hours went by and evening darkened the shadows in the corners of the room.

Rolling over, Elizabeth woke to a noise. She had to orient herself to the time of day as well as the date. As she slowly came to consciousness, she continued to hear a noise from the living room. Reaching out, she turned the nightstand light on. She sat for a minute to make sure she wasn't dizzy and then walked to the bathroom.

After washing her hands, she strode toward the kitchen and stopped when she realized there was a banging on her front door. Fear enveloped her as she wasn't expecting anyone, including herself, to be home during the day or early evening. Slowly she went to the door, stood on her toes to peek through the eyepiece and relaxed when she saw Jake at the door.

He continued to knock as he called out. "Elizabeth, are you in there? Elizabeth, open the door." He pulled out his cell phone and was about to call the station when he heard the door click open.

She stood there, recent sleep written over her face, her hair askew from the pillow.

"Jake?"

He looked her over before responding. "Are you okay?"

Elizabeth combed her hair with her fingers as she stepped back and opened the door to allow him to enter. "Sure, c'mon inside."

"Are you sick? It's early evening."

"No, I just had a bit of a meltdown so I came home to get some sleep."

"Do you feel better?"

Elizabeth stopped to think for a moment. "Yes, I think I do. It was one of those deep sleeps where you don't dream, you don't move, you just sleep." Frank hadn't appeared and for the first time she questioned why he hadn't.

"Did anything specific happen today?"

Elizabeth's stomach gurgled. "Listen, let me brush my hair and we'll talk about it."

"I'm going to assume you haven't eaten anything so grab a jacket and we'll talk over a meal. I'll drive." Jake held up his keys.

Nodding, Elizabeth quietly went into her bedroom while Jake waited near the door. He looked around her condo while he stood there.

Her place was neat as a pin. The condo was modern, comfortable and well decorated, but it wasn't flashy and didn't have expensive art scattered about for effect. She had a large bookcase along the far wall filled with books. He hoped he'd have the opportunity to explore her favorite titles.

"Okay, I'm ready," Elizabeth said as she came from the bedroom.

She had brushed her hair and washed her face. Jake admired her natural beauty. She didn't need make-up to be beautiful.

After Elizabeth locked her doors, the two walked down to Jake's car. He opened the passenger door and waited until she was seated in the spotless Ford Crown Victoria.

"Are you comfortable?" Jake asked as he handed her the seat belt.

"Yes, I'm good. Thank you."

Jake went around the car and got into the driver's side. He belted himself in and turned onto the main road.

"Where are we going?" Elizabeth asked as she turned toward him. "I'm hungry but not dressed to go anywhere."

"Not to worry. I've got a great little casual fun place to eat when you don't want fancy."

"Sounds interesting."

"You like Latin music?"

"Most of it, yes. I like other types of music as well."

"Such as?"

"I like Country Reggae, you know beach music like Jimmy Buffett and Kenny Chesney. How about you?"

"I like Jazz, but a lot of other stuff, too. Have you been to the New Wales Park lately? The one near the Hudson River?"

"Not in a long while," Elizabeth said as Jake turned into the park and found a parking space.

"Then you're in for a treat. The food trucks are here for another hour. I know it sounds low rent, but it's a great place."

Elizabeth got out of the car and walked with Jake down a concrete path along the Hudson River. The park was beautiful, especially under the lights at night. At the far end, several food trucks were parked and each had a significant line of people waiting to place their order. When she turned to look at the Hudson, the magnificent view of the Manhattan evening skyline loomed before her. The lights had a way of making the city twinkle like magic.

"Beautiful, isn't it?" Jake was watching her reaction to the view.

"It really is," Elizabeth said. "Between going to the hospital and home, I haven't come to the park for many years. I've never seen it look this beautiful. They've done a lot of renovation since I've been here."

"It's a great place, day or night," Jake said.

"Isn't it amazing how alive the city looks at night? Especially from a distance, the lights are beautiful."

"There's a lot of excitement there," Jake said as he listened to Elizabeth's stomach growl. "C'mon, let's get something to eat. You like Mexican food?"

"Sure do."

"Then, we're going to Poppi's. I guarantee you'll have the best taco and burrito you've ever eaten."

"Okay, I'll let you order."

The pair reached Poppi's food truck. They waited on line for a short time and when they reached the window, Jake ordered for them. They were given a paper boat filled with tortilla chips as well as another with small plastic cups of salsa and queso. Munching on their chips, they stood near the truck and waited for their order. When it was ready, they found their way over to a group of picnic tables, under some trees, near the Hudson.

"Well, what do you think?" Jake asked, watching her bite into the taco.

Elizabeth finished chewing. "This is delicious. Better than a lot of restaurants I've been to."

"You bet. Poppi's is the best." They continued to eat until they were full, enjoying the breeze and temperate night air.

Pushing back the paper boat and crumpling the paper, Elizabeth sat up straight. "That was delicious. Thank you."

Jake laughed. "Don't thank me yet. I still plan on asking you what happened today."

Elizabeth shrugged her shoulders as she continued to watch the reflection of the city lights in the river.

"C'mon, time to tell me the truth. I'm on your side here. You've gotta know that by now."

Elizabeth started to speak. At first her works were soft, but then gained strength as she vented.

"I've been very stressed since these patients died. I've been over it again and again and I've been reviewed, but my surgical technique was fine. As you know, the death of these two patients were from weird complications. The types of vessel rupture they died from was not apparent on the CT scans prior to the surgery."

"Regardless, Dr. Pruitt, who is the Department Chairman has been after me, harassing me, as if single-handedly, I've been the only surgeon to lose a patient."

"The autopsy report I read didn't say anything about physician error or technique."

Elizabeth shook her head. "Because there was none. I've now heard about a couple of other problems and I think it all traces back to this MemorHold. Dr. Pruitt just had one of his surgical patients die. At first, the chart didn't say anything about the supplement but the hand written list of meds that the patient brought with him has MemorHold listed."

"What did Pruitt have to say about that?"

"That's just it. After months of harassment, being pulled into department review, having a lawsuit slapped on me, and old fashioned arrogance and bullying, I told him what I thought today. I told him about MemorHold and I told him I reported it to the FDA Safety Portal."

"You reported it?"

Elizabeth nodded. "I did. I had my charts audited. I audited the charts of the patients who died and they all have that common link."

"Did you tell Pruitt?"

"I did and he went absolutely apoplectic. I told him he should check his charts. I didn't look at his specifically. He turned purple, his neck veins bulged and he was screaming at me in the middle of the café. Everyone heard him."

"Why would he do that?" Jake asked as he stared at her.

"Because he doesn't want the deaths to be a result of a medication or a supply problem. He wants it to be because of me so he can ditch me. Also, my making that complaint will definitely bring investigators to the hospital to review our program. He'll have to justify everything that goes on there. He doesn't like having female surgeons on staff. Pruitt has always been part of the good-old boy club. He can't tolerate woman in the field, his field anyway."

"The guy knows we're in the twenty-first century right?" Jake asked.

"We are, but I don't think he ever progressed. Anyway, when I pointed out that his patient might have died for the same reason, he lost it. First of all, he doesn't want to admit he lost a patient at all. I gave him an out, but that wasn't good enough. He has two sets of standards. One for him and his buddies and another for me."

Jake stared at her as she spoke and noticed how beautiful she looked. "So now what?"

"Well, I realized, after the fact, that I just pulled the problem into the cross hairs. At some point, your buddy Phil is going to get a call from the FDA and they'll hopefully start an investigation. That will lead them to the hospital to look at my deaths which I'll have to defend. They will also ask about the death of Dr. Pruitt's patient so he'll have to speak to that. If he acknowledges the link to MemorHold to save his reputation, he loses his argument against my privileges and surgical technique before the board. I put him between a rock and hard place."

"That's interesting. What did you mean when you said, 'my buddy, Phil?"

"I didn't really mean your buddy. I was being sarcastic since I know you went and spoke to him."

Jake paused and looked at Elizabeth.

"What's wrong?" She asked when she saw his facial expression.

"How did you know I spoke with Phil?"

"You told me, didn't you?"

"No, I haven't had a chance to tell you about the investigation."

"Well, you did talk to him, right?"

"Yes, but that's beside the point. How did you know?"

Elizabeth's face reddened when she realized the person who told her was Frank. She couldn't admit that to anyone otherwise they'd think she truly was crazy. "I'm pretty sure you mentioned you were going to talk to him."

"I did, but you had no way of knowing we went. Are you sure you didn't speak to someone?" Jake was confused. He was so sure Elizabeth was an innocent victim in this mess, but now he wondered. He had specifically looked around her waiting room the first time he made an appointment and noticed she wasn't selling any supplements or even pushing fliers about them. How could she have known he went and spoke to Phil? Although he hated to admit it, he'd have to go back again and make sure there was no connection with Phil in her history. He needed to make sure they didn't go to college together or have an old relationship.

"Earth to Jake. Are you still in there?"

Jake shook his head. "I'm sorry. What did you say?"

Elizabeth was annoyed. "I don't know because I'm not sure where you checked out."

Jake apologized again. "I was just making some connections in my head. So tell me again, how did you come to be home today?"

Elizabeth took a deep breath. "It's a good thing you bought me dinner. After my altercation with Pruitt, I went into the bathroom. Caitlyn followed me and it's a good thing she did, because I was starting to have a panic attack. She's the one who pushed me to go the hell home and get some sleep. She told me to get out before anything else happened and for once, I listened to her. I was exhausted."

"And you went straight home?" Jake asked as he made a note to speak to Caitlyn.

"I sure did. I thought I'd take a nap but I wound up sleeping for hours and the next thing I knew, you were at my door."

Jake nodded his understanding. "Caitlyn is protective of you."

"Yes, she is and I should be more thankful. By the way, thank you for making sure I had a good meal. I appreciate the company since it was such a lousy day."

"My pleasure," Jake said softly. He stood up, threw everything in the garbage and grabbed Elizabeth by the hand. "C'mon, let's walk along the river and enjoy the sights."

# CHAPTER 49

Elizabeth woke the next morning to sunlight. She slept well which was surprising considering she had slept at length the day before. Frank hadn't appeared last night. Maybe she was crazy and Frank was a manifestation of her insomnia and sleep deprivation.

She enjoyed her time with Jake, perhaps that helped her relax and sleep better. After their walk, he drove her home and made sure she was locked up safe in the condo. A small warning bell went off in her mind that she shouldn't get used to having him around. He would most likely be gone as soon as this business was straightened out.

Elizabeth dressed, had a quick cup of coffee and was on her way to the hospital when her cell phone rang. The caller ID in her car indicated the caller was Heather. Elizabeth punched the green icon on her car touch screen.

"Good morning, Heather. What's up?"

"It's not that good of a morning. You'd better get over here right away."

"I'm on my way to the hospital to see Mr. Jackson. Saturday morning rounds are usually pretty quick."

"No, you need to be here now. The police are on their way." Heather hung up the phone as Elizabeth's chest constricted.

She punched the accelerator and flew to her office. What the hell happened that the police would have to be there? There were no patients scheduled yet. Luckily, no one was monitoring radar as she sped to the office. She pulled into the parking lot and saw several police cars as well as Jake's Crown Victoria. There were officers walking about. On the side of the parking lot, she saw Heather with some of the weekend staff as well as a few of the morning patients.

Elizabeth quickly parked and jumped out of her car. She ran to the front of the building to figure out what was going on. After a minute, she walked to Heather to get more information.

"What happened?"

"Someone broke into your office last night," Heather said, upset and shaken.

Elizabeth turned to see the front door of the office was broken as well as one of the front windows. "Someone looking for drugs?"

She stopped speaking when she saw Jake walk toward her with a grim look on his face. She walked up to meet him. "What's going on?"

"You've had a visitor but this was no random break-in."

"How do you know?"

He reached out and took her by the arm. "You'd better come with me." He escorted her to the front door, broken glass was all over the ground as well as inside on the carpet and scattered into the waiting area. Chairs in the waiting room were toppled and slashed. The knob to the inner office had been broken off and the door hung open.

"I need you to look everything over without touching a thing," Jake said as he walked her through the office. "You'll know best if anything is missing and I want you to see what destruction has been done and let me know what it means."

Elizabeth stared up at him. "Okay, but you're frightening me."

"That's not my intent. That's why I'm doing the walk through with you. We'll just go room by room."

"Okay." The pair slowly walked down the hall and noted each exam room had items strewn all over the floors. The naugahyde on the exam tables had been slashed. Elizabeth was upset by everything she saw but she gasped when she went into her office.

"Take your time, but don't touch anything," Jake said, watching her closely.

Close to tears, Elizabeth was speechless. Everything on her desk was ripped up and thrown all over. Her desk was toppled. Her frames were smashed. Her books were all over the floor and the bookcase pushed over. But the worst thing was someone had spray painted over her wall. Red paint, looking very much like blood, dripped down the wall, and spelled out,

*You're going to Pay!!!!*

ELIZABETH'S HANDS flew to her mouth. "Oh, no. Who would do this?"

Jake put his arm around her as she started to shake. "That's what we have to talk about. Just breathe. Slow deep breaths." He then pulled her into a full body hug. Feeling his strong warmth around her, she calmed down. She felt better and didn't want to move but she pushed back and looked up at Jake.

"Thank you for being here. I just can't believe someone would do something so evil."

"You'd be surprised. I don't want to get you upset again but what's the first name that comes to your mind?"

Elizabeth shook her head side to side. "The most obvious thing I can think of is that the FDA paid MemorHold a visit or called for records."

"Have you had any other threats or angry patients?"

Taking a moment to think, Elizabeth said, "No, except I'm being sued by Frank Burdette's family. But why would they do something like this now? It's been months and they already filed the suit."

"Grief is a funny thing," Jake said.

"No, it doesn't make sense."

Jake turned her to face him. "I want you to go through all your medicine cabinets. Check your logs for drugs. Let's find out if anything is missing. Have you had a patient you recently refused meds to?"

"Are you kidding me? With the new laws, I refuse narcotic prescriptions every day. I had a patient who recently demanded I give him a bottle of morphine but I refused. I sent him to a pain clinic. I have several patients that are registered to the local methadone clinic but there have never been any problems with those patients. As a matter of fact, they're some of the more respectful patients."

"Someone is angry with you, that's quite evident."

"I'd suggest you go back to your friend, Phil, and ask him. I know he wouldn't get his hands dirty, but I'm sure he could easily get someone to come in here and do this, especially if they thought there were drugs available."

"We're collecting evidence now. First, I'd like to gather more information. Is there any chance you have cameras or video of your office?"

"I don't have any video near the exam rooms due to privacy. We do have a camera on the parking lot. We have a security company that monitors our alarm and video."

"That's interesting. There was no report called in and this damage didn't happen in five minutes. It wasn't picked up until your nurse Heather arrived at the building this morning."

Shaking her head, Elizabeth said, "I have no idea. I should talk to Heather. We have patients waiting in the parking lot. Obviously, we have to send everyone home and cancel the appointments. I'll have to speak with the practice manager. They'll probably have the patients go to another office."

"What do you mean, the practice manager? Explain that to me. Here, you'd better sit down. You look pale. I'll send an officer to bring Heather inside."

Elizabeth wearily sat in a chair that hadn't been toppled. When Jake returned a moment later, she said, "This practice is owned by the hospital. They own most of the doctor's offices so they manage them. The doctors are given a schedule of hours and we work for a salary just like everyone else. So the destruction is not necessarily about me as it may be about the hospital in general."

"Or it may be directly related to you," Jake pointed out.

"Yes, I guess that's true," Elizabeth said as she looked at him. "Anyway, they own the building and the practice so I need to call someone in the management group. They'll arrange for the office repair and reschedule the patients to another office until this office is cleared."

Hearing a knock, the pair turned to see Heather and an officer standing near the door. Elizabeth jumped up and went over to hug Heather. "Are you okay? I can't believe you walked into this mess."

"I didn't go inside. I called the police as soon as I saw the broken front door." Heather jumped when she read the words spray-painted on the wall.

"What's that all about?"

"Who knows? Heather, was there an alarm going off when you got here?"

"No, nothing which is why I was surprised. I thought the vandals broke it."

"Did you call the practice manager yet?" Elizabeth asked while looking around.

"No, but we'd better get to it."

Elizabeth turned toward Jake. "Can we call them?"

"Sure," Jake said. "Maybe it will help straighten this out. What about appointment books or charts?"

"Most of our information, including patient records and appointment scheduling is on the main system so it can be accessed at any computer. We can go to another office. When can we start picking up this place?"

Jake looked at the officer who shook his head. "Apparently, we still have some processing to do. We'll call you and let you know."

"I guess that's best. They may want an insurance company representative to take a look before they do anything," Elizabeth said.

"Why don't the two of you go outside and make your call? Let me know what they say and then we'll regroup."

"Okay." Elizabeth and Heather followed the officer to the front door and went to sit in Elizabeth's car while they called.

Alex walked into Elizabeth's office as the two women walked out. "So, what do you think?"

Jake shook his head. "I think she was not only surprised, she was scared. This was a shock for her. Have you found anything useful yet?"

"No," Alex said. "I don't think anything was taken. It's clearly a message to Elizabeth. I know we talked last night about this but I'm going to ask again. Are you sure you can trust her? Are you sure she's not involved somehow?"

"I'll admit, I still want to know how she knew we went to see Phil Harry at MemorHold. There's only two ways she could have found out. Either through Phil or his little Administrative Assistant."

"That's interesting," Alex said. "Maybe the assistant is a patient of Dr. Brooks's?"

"She could be her sister for all I know," Jake said. "But I believe you're going to let your fingers do the walking and see if there's any relationship? Check all the phone records. See if Elizabeth received any calls from anyone at MemorHold recently and cross check with her friend, Caitlyn, as well. Make sure she doesn't have any ties with anyone at the company."

"You've got it," Alex said.

They turned when they heard voices. Elizabeth, Heather and the officer were back.

"Did you get hold of the management?" Jake asked.

"Yes, we did," Elizabeth said. "First of all, the representative said they were converting the security system so they apologized but there was no security last night."

"No kidding?" Jake asked, eyebrows raised as he looked at Alex.

Elizabeth caught their exchange and her eyes set. "No, no kidding. He actually said that's bad for them because the insurance company could refuse the claim. Having the alarm set is part of the policy protocol."

Alex nodded. "I imagine so."

Turning to Alex, Elizabeth said, "You were right. The insurance agent will want to come over before anything is cleaned up. He's on his way over right now. Once they're done, they'll make arrangements for someone to come over and start cleaning the place as soon as you clear it.

"What about you in the meantime?" Jake asked.

"I still have to go to the hospital and do rounds. Heather will go to the office on Main Street and call the patients."

"Before you do that, can we take a quick tour of the office to see if you think anything is missing?"

"Sure, let's go."

The four of them went into each room. Elizabeth and Heather told them what to look for. Alex used a pencil to sort through drawers and cabinets to not leave any fingerprints. They took extra time to look through the business office. Although everything was a mess, it didn't appear that anything was missing. There was no money in the office as everything from the week had been deposited the night before. They ended up near the front door.

Both Heather and Elizabeth voiced their schedules for the remainder of the day and made arrangements to leave. As Elizabeth got into her car, Jake quickly ran over and looked in the driver's window.

"Hey, I was just thinking. Make sure you keep your cell phone close and I'll give you a call later. Just in case you think of something or anything happens, call me directly."

"Okay," Elizabeth said as she inwardly berated herself. It took an event like this to get a man to call her. The fact that he was incredibly handsome had nothing to do with it. "Jake, I'm scared. Please find out who did this."

"I promise I will. Be careful out there today. Don't go anywhere alone and call me if you see anything suspicious at all."

"Will do," she said with a small smile as she held up her phone. "I'd better get to the hospital."

Jake stepped back, checked the parking lot for pedestrians and tapped the roof of the car. He watched as she backed out of the space and sped away.

# CHAPTER 50

Elizabeth drove toward the hospital. She told herself she was fine, but she could feel herself shaking inside. It was unbelievable that someone would do that much damage. She parked in the parking garage and went into the hospital through the surgical locker room. She put her things in her locker and went to make rounds. Mr. Jackson had been moved into a regular room and was looking well. He'd be ready for discharge soon.

Elizabeth checked his chart once again to confirm his final biopsy did return with a benign diagnosis. His lab and exams looked great. As she readied to leave his room, he thanked her once again. "Take care of yourself, Doc. Be careful." She turned and asked him to repeat what he said. Shrugging, he said, "Just saying goodbye."

Walking back to the surgical suite, she finished her note, checked her schedule for OR time and went to get her things from her locker. As she walked past a group of clinicians at the nurses's desk, she heard her name called out.

"Brooks."

She turned around to find that Dr. Pruitt was calling her. She immediately tensed when she saw him staring at her.

"Yes, Dr. Pruitt?" She stopped without smiling and waited for him to continue.

"I, ah, apparently owe you an apology."

"Say what?" Elizabeth asked, incredulous.

"Our conversation was overheard by our CEO in the lunchroom the other day and I've been instructed to apologize to you immediately."

Elizabeth smiled as she knew he must be having chest pain as he carried out his forced apology. "Why, thank you Dr. Pruitt. Hopefully, we can establish a better working relationship in the future."

The clinicians around them had all gone silent as they realized they were witnessing a historic apology from Pruitt.

He nodded slightly. "Perhaps that will happen. The hospital administration wants to make sure you understand that our discussion and my response in no way reflect the type of behavior they condone here."

"I understand, and thank you. Good day, Dr. Pruitt." Elizabeth turned to leave when he called her back.

"If our illustrious CEO calls, you'll be sure to tell him we had this conversation."

She now understood he purposely apologized in front of the nurses in order to have witnesses.

"Of course, thank you." Elizabeth left the surgical locker room and scurried to her car. She shook off the willies. Having him apologize was worse than when he yelled. Backing out of her parking space, she left the hospital and drove to her office. Most of the police cars had left. Only one patrol and a plain car remained. Elizabeth parked and walked up to the officer at the door. "Hi, I'm Dr. Brooks. I'm just checking to see if you found anything specific?"

The officer recognized her and smiled politely. "I can't talk about an on-going investigation ma'am."

Elizabeth winced inwardly at his words. She wasn't old enough to be a ma'am or was she?

"I can't let you in here, either."

"That's okay, I didn't ask to go in. I just wanted to know if there was any progress."

The young officer shrugged and smiled. Elizabeth thanked him and returned to her car. She called Heather and asked about her progress with the appointments.

"I'm just about done. The patients understood and feel bad about the office. One or two were upset and screaming how the only day they can come to the office was on a Saturday, so we brought them into the Main Street office and had Dr. Hadley take care of them. I've rescheduled everyone up to Wednesday and I'll finish the rest of the week before I go home."

"Thanks, Heather. You're the best."

"Well, the only problem is you were scheduled to see Lucky, on Monday. I had to cancel his appointment because he wasn't able to get a bus for this office. He has another appointment in four weeks but he said he's feeling okay."

"Okay, maybe we can call and check on him in a week or so to make sure he's still doing well."

"You've got it, boss."

"Thanks again. I'm going to do some paperwork at home. If you need me, please call anytime."

"Will do, thanks, Doc Brooks."

"For what? Just take care of yourself and once again I'm sorry you had to walk into that mess. It must have been scary."

"Yes, it was, but I'm doing fine." She hesitated. "Will you be okay? I'm a little worried about what was written on the wall."

"I'm fine, but do me a favor and let's try to keep that little detail private. I don't think we want to create any anxiety for the patients."

"Just you and me, Doc. I promise."

"I believe you," Elizabeth said. "Talk to you soon."

# CHAPTER 51

Elizabeth spent the afternoon reading lab reports and reviewing office charts from the computer in her condo. Her mind wandered as she worked. Three times she picked up the phone. She wanted to call Jake and find out what he'd done so far. Most of all, she wanted to know if he went and found that scum Phil Harry. She was so mad, she wanted to go down there and punch his lights out herself.

Elizabeth pushed on with her paperwork until she was done. Stretching, she padded to the kitchen and made herself a sandwich. She added an apple to the plate and poured herself a glass of water. Picking up the remote, she put on the news. The usual interest stories about assault and robbery, drugs, politics, weather and traffic were featured. Next came a feature about a destructive break-in at a doctor's office. Elizabeth stiffened when she saw aerial coverage of her office. She listened closely as the announcers discussed the police response. There was no real information other than the fact there was a break-in and of course, her name was mentioned on the news. Just then, her cell phone buzzed.

Elizabeth saw the number on the phone and didn't answer as she didn't recognize it. It was mere seconds before the phone rang again with a different number. Her phone continued to ring on and off for a full ten minutes. When she saw Jake's number on the caller ID, she answered immediately.

"Jake? I don't believe it," Elizabeth said.

"I take it you saw the news."

"My phone has not stopped ringing for ten minutes. I'm ignoring all calls because I have no idea who they're from or how they got my number and I don't want to be asked for a statement. I didn't see any news vans when I was there."

"They swooped in after you left," Jake said. "Anyone can make a statement. They could have called a patient, a nurse, who knows."

"How did they get the aerial footage?"

"A drone. All the newsrooms have them now. Hell of a lot cheaper than sending up a helicopter every day."

"I can't believe they can invade your privacy like that."

"Well, believe it. How did the rest of your day go? Any problems?"

"It was fine. I did rounds at the hospital and then went home. I stopped back at the office, but a very young, polite officer sent me packing."

Jake chuckled. "Be glad he did. If he wasn't there, you probably would have had reporters taking inside photos of the office."

"I wasn't happy at the time, but now I get it," Elizabeth said. "Did you find anything today? Any idea who did this or why?"

"Nothing specific yet. We'll wait for prints but I wouldn't get excited."

"There must be a thousand sets of prints from all the patients."

"Yes, there's that," Jake said. "Did you hear anything else from the management company or insurance company?"

"No, not beyond the initial notification," Elizabeth said. "Why do you ask?"

"One of the reasons I'm calling is to tell you that the police have what they need from the building. The scene will be released in the morning so you or your management company or insurance company are free to do whatever you want."

"Oh, great. I need to call them and see what they're doing. I'm not sure if the insurance representative is done. Then I need to know how they plan to clean it up and how much we need to do ourselves. I'll go down there tomorrow and start picking through the rubble. They'll deal with the furniture and locks but I want to see what state the records are in."

"That certainly sounds like a plan. I'll probably stop by and see how you're doing at some point late tomorrow morning."

"Okay, great. Thanks," Elizabeth said, pleased that she would see him although she'd never let him know that.

"As a matter of fact, call your management and insurance agents and then let me know when you're going. I'll meet you down there and make sure it's safe before you go in."

"Thank you, Jake. That's very sweet of you. I'll touch base in the morning, I promise," Elizabeth said.

"Okay, try to get some rest tonight. Try not to think about about it."

Elizabeth laughed. "If you only knew about my sleep habits. They're not great on a good day."

"Maybe I'll find out first-hand one day," Jake said.

Elizabeth's face flamed red as her eyes opened wide. "Hmm." She hung her head thinking of a way not to say something stupid and so very glad he couldn't see her right now.

"Are all your doors and windows locked?"

"I think so," she said, although not really sure.

"Go lock everything. I'll hang on until you do."

"Are you sure? That could take a while."

"Yes, go do it, now," Jake instructed.

"Okay, please hold," Elizabeth teased as she put the phone down. She spent ten minutes visiting all doors and windows and realized the condo was not locked up. She had started working in daylight and wasn't concerned then. Day had turned into night and she hadn't thought of locking up.

"Everything is now tightly secured," Elizabeth said as she returned to the phone.

"Good, sleep tight, Elizabeth. I'll see you tomorrow."

"Goodnight, Jake," Elizabeth said softly as she hung up the phone. Her voice had quivered a bit and she hoped he didn't hear that. He would probably be laughing if he realized his effect on her.

Elizabeth's face continued to flame as she thought of his words and the butterflies in her stomach when she thought of his touch. He was so charming and attractive, she couldn't imagine why he didn't have ten women hanging over him, begging for attention. More likely, there was something drastically wrong with him and she just hadn't found out what it was yet. Otherwise, he would have been married for ten years and have four children at home with a wife. Elizabeth began to get sleepy as she laughed to herself. For all she knew, he did have a wife and family at home.

# CHAPTER 52

*She was walking toward the trees. She couldn't see any sunlight or reflection through the leaves. The wind was blowing and the trees were swaying in a macabre dance. Elizabeth wasn't sure why, but she felt alone. She looked for Frank, but didn't see him anywhere. She felt nervous and ran forward looking toward the shed.*

*Elizabeth called out Frank's name but was not met with an answer. She didn't understand it. Where did he go? Why would he leave her now? The shed appeared in the distance and Elizabeth ran toward it. Cold, thick raindrops pelted her face, her head and body. Elizabeth ran faster.*

*When she reached the shed she flung open the door and stepped inside. The shed smelled of freshly mowed grass and hay. "Frank? Are you here?" She looked around but didn't see anyone. "Frank? You're scaring me."*

*Elizabeth spun when she heard a voice from the corner of the shed. "You need to be careful now."*

*"Connie?" Elizabeth blinked as she saw the image of Connie Arturo standing next to Frank. She wasn't as solid as Frank and appeared anxious. "Frank?"*

*"You have to be careful, watch your back. We had to come to you."*

*"Can anyone come to me who wants to?" Elizabeth asked.*

*Frank shook his head. "It's complicated. It's the expected and unexpected."*

*"What are you saying? I don't understand."*

*"We have to go," Frank said as Connie took a few steps toward Elizabeth. "Please do me a favor. Go to Pasquale. Tell him to look behind the credenza. Pull it out and look for an envelope. Tell him, to give the envelope to the police. I have to go. Tell him," Connie said as her voice and visage faded right in front of Elizabeth. The wind roared around the shed and seconds later the door blew open and banged against the wall.*

ELIZABETH JUMPED when she heard the door bang. She sat for a few moments. She was sure she heard a door bang. Was it the dream or did she really hear a door? Rubbing the back of her neck, she'd have to talk to someone soon. Was she having contact with the beyond or was her brain working out her problems?

Shaking, she stood up and went to the threshold of her bedroom. She stood quietly, listening, trying to make shapes out of the shadows. The ticking of the clock was deafening. She was probably one of the last people who had a clock with moving parts hanging on the wall but she refused to go completely digital. Ten minutes went by and she heard nothing unusual.

Elizabeth turned on a small lamp in the hall and once again strained to listen for any strange noises. At the moment, she wished Jake was staying the night with her, but for different reasons than he probably wanted.

After a few minutes, she was brave enough to go downstairs to the living room and turn on a few lamps. She made her way through the condo, rechecking doors and windows and found everything was locked.

Chiding herself, she decided to go back to bed. She went upstairs but left the lights on. Had she looked out the window, she may have seen a Crown Victoria parked halfway down the street.

# CHAPTER 53

Elizabeth opened her eyes the next morning to sunlight. It had taken an hour to fall back to sleep after her dream and search for intruders. She knew she heard a door slam but couldn't be sure if it was part of the dream or her condo. Since she was still alive and slept the rest of the night she assumed it was the dream after all.

Rolling out of bed, she headed for the shower. After allowing the hot steam to relax her muscles, she dried off, dressed and headed downstairs. She put on a full pot of coffee and waited for the rich, dark liquid to be ready to pour into her cup. As she was deciding what to do for breakfast, she heard a knock on the door. She peeked through the window before she opened it.

"Mom, Dad, what are you doing here so early?" Elizabeth didn't have time for the answer as Goldy pulled the leash out of Parker's hand, scrabbled over the threshold and jumped on Elizabeth. She immediately dropped to one knee and hugged the dog, scratched her head and received unrelenting kisses in return.

"Goldy, you are the sweetest girl."

"Parker, why did you let her go like that?" C.J. asked.

"I didn't let her go, she ran the minute she saw Lizzie. As a matter of fact, she was excited before Lizzie opened the door. I think she knew where we were."

"That's impossible, she's never been here before."

Parker shrugged. "What do I know? Maybe she smelled her."

Elizabeth tried again. "I didn't expect you guys so early."

"I'm surprised we made it at all," Parker said. "You're mother must have hit every pothole between the shore and here. Actually, she missed one so I asked her if she wanted to go home and try it again."

C.J. walked past Elizabeth carrying a bag of groceries. She rolled her eyes as she put the bag on the kitchen table. "Oh good, you haven't eaten yet. I was afraid we'd be too late."

"No, I just got up," Elizabeth said. "Not that it's any surprise, but I didn't sleep well the first half of the night, so I slept in."

"The coffee smells great," Parker said as he walked inside.

"Well, that's better for us. We bought everything for an old fashioned breakfast. Eggs, bacon, pancakes and orange juice. Your favorite since you were a little girl."

Elizabeth played with Goldy in the living room. When they took a break, Elizabeth found a plastic dish and filled it with water for her. After the dog drank most of the cool water, she pulled Elizabeth down and started licking her face again.

"I'm so happy you brought Goldy with you," Elizabeth said.

"I have news for you, she wasn't going to have it any other way. I'm telling you the dog knew we were going to visit and insisted she be in the car before any of us."

Elizabeth hugged her again. "Aw, aren't you the most beautiful dog?"

"Honey, why don't you take her for a walk around the yard while your father and I make breakfast?"

Elizabeth looked at her parents and realized it would be best to be out of their way. She put on her running shoes and picked up Goldy's leash. The pair went out the door and trotted toward the small park a couple of blocks away. They maintained an even pace until they approached the park. Goldy stopped short and growled.

"What is it, girl? What's wrong?"

Elizabeth looked up and saw a few children in the park and a couple of people walking down the street. A man sat near the park in his car and Goldy barked at him until he closed the driver's side door.

"Goldy, stop that or I'll have to bring you home." They continued their trot, passing other walkers and the children in the park. Goldy smiled and seemed happy to be out and about.

Circling the block, they returned back to her condo and went inside. Her father had finished making the bacon, while her mother whipped up the eggs and pancakes. The table was set for the three of them.

While Goldy lapped up more cool water, Elizabeth pulled three mugs out of the cabinet for coffee and glasses for the juice.

"How was your walk?" C.J. asked as she continued flipping pancakes.

"It was great until Goldy saw a man in the park. She didn't like him because she growled and snarled until he got in his car."

"Really?" Parker asked, as he plated a few pieces of bacon. "That's strange, because she's usually pretty friendly."

"She didn't like this guy. I've heard it said that dogs are a good test of character, so if she didn't like him, she may know more than us."

"Could very well be," C.J. said. "Let's sit down and eat."

The group passed the food plates and saved a few small pieces for Goldy. "Delicious. You always make a great breakfast together."

"I couldn't find any strawberries, but maybe next time," C.J. said as she buttered her pancake.

"So, what do you have in mind to do today?" Parker finished his coffee and poured a little more into his cup.

Elizabeth paused before she answered. "I didn't realize you were coming so early. I had a little problem yesterday and I have to go work on it."

"Oh really, like the vandalism at your office?" Parker popped another piece of bacon in his mouth.

"You saw it on the news?" Elizabeth asked.

"Even if we didn't, we would have figured it out by the multitude of phone calls we received after it was reported."

"I'm sorry. I should have called you," Elizabeth said.

"What exactly happened yesterday, Lizzie?"

Elizabeth put her fork down. "I was on my way to the hospital and I got a call from Heather to come to the office immediately. She didn't tell me why except the police were there. When I got there, they showed me the vandalism and escorted me through the office to see if anything had been stolen." Elizabeth looked at her father. "The entire office was destroyed. Chairs turned over, tables were slashed, locks broken off the doors and other things." Elizabeth stopped talking when she saw the look on her mother's face.

"Do the police have any leads?" Parker asked.

"They didn't offer an opinion other than they'll start an investigation. We talked about possibilities, but that's it. I was planning to go to the office after my coffee this morning. I thought you'd be here later in the day. The detective called me last night and told me they cleared the scene for cleaning but I have to call management to see if it's okay."

Parker swallowed more coffee and nodded. "That's fine, you go ahead and make your calls while we clean up. Do you have any idea who would be angry enough to do that sort of thing?"

"Dad, I told you my patients were on MemorHold. Also, from what John Donovan said about the problems with vascular weakness, I'll bet those patients were taking the supplement as well, so I reported it to the FDA Safety Portal a couple of days ago. I tried to make the claim anonymously, but apparently I didn't get it right. I'm thinking, they may have gotten a call or visit from the FDA."

"It's possible," Parker said. "But that would be the fastest government response I ever saw."

"I know," Elizabeth said, "But that's all I can think of."

C.J. stood and collected the plates and utensils off the table. Goldy whimpered and placed her head on Elizabeth's leg.

"Why don't you make your phone call and then we'll talk about going down there."

"Okay, Jake will be there. Maybe, he'll have more information for us."

"Jake?" C.J. asked as she turned toward her daughter.

"The lead detective on the case. His name is Jake Wagner. It's confusing because Jake was already investigating the company for embezzlement when my first patient, who turned out to be the CFO for the company, unexpectedly died on me. Jake was originally looking for a connection between the two, but the surgical death was not connected."

Parker picked up his mug and drank. "It would certainly be Karma to steal from your company and then pass away before you were able to enjoy the money."

"Yes," Elizabeth agreed, "but what's worse is that my second patient who died this year happened to be the first patient's coworker. She also worked for the same department. So now, the detective, Jake, is looking at two people who may have embezzled and then both mysteriously died. Obviously, he was looking at all angles and thought I was involved."

"Technically, you are involved, just not for any reason he's looking for."

"I'm sure he and his partner have now clawed through whatever data they can find about me. If they looked at my bank accounts, I'm sure they weren't impressed." Elizabeth chuckled at her statement."Initially, I was angry and ditched him at every turn, but I figured I could find out more information if I cooperated. Any information could only help my case."

"True, but it may be better if you let the professionals take care of the matter," C.J. said. "Being so close to this break-in and dead people scares me."

"Lizzie, why don't you go and make your phone call so we can clean up and then we'll make plans."

Elizabeth stood up and gave her parents a peck on their cheeks. "Okay, thanks for breakfast. Hopefully, I'll be right back."

She picked up her cell phone and went into the living room. Parker called to Goldy, but the dog followed Elizabeth and wouldn't leave her side. When Elizabeth sat on the couch, Goldy jumped up and placed her head on Elizabeth's lap, with her paw across Elizabeth's leg.

Elizabeth chuckled. "Awww. I'm okay, girl. You don't have to worry, but thank you for your company." She punched up her contacts and dialed the management company. After several rings, she was able to speak to the representative who advised her the insurance company had already finished their appraisal and she could go to the office to check for personal items. She was advised that someone had been dispatched to start repair on the exam tables and door locks, but it would take a few days to fix. The office would remain closed for the week and the patients would be rerouted to the Main Street office until repairs were made. Elizabeth was expected to examine her patients in the alternate office until then.

"Thank you," Elizabeth said as she hung up the phone.

"Well, how did it go?" Parker asked as he wandered into the living room. He had a towel in his hands and was drying a dish as he spoke.

"They're all over it," Elizabeth said with a sarcastic frown. "They already have a crew doing repairs. I can check for personal things but I should be ready bright and early Monday morning to see my patients in an alternate location."

Parker walked to his daughter and gave her a hug. "Medicine has changed drastically over the last thirty years. I'm sorry they treat you that way."

"They're taking care of everything but it all sounds so cold and sterile." Elizabeth mocked them. 'You'll report here and do this there.' I wanted to shout at them. The only person who asked if I was okay was Jake, except for you and mom."

C.J. walked over and joined the group hug while Goldy danced at their feet. "C'mon, let's go over there and make sure your stuff is all intact. Your father and I are not leaving your side."

"Thank you," Elizabeth said. "Do you want to take my car?"

"As long as you don't mind Goldy being in there because she's not going to let you leave without her."

"That's fine. Goldy is welcome in my car."

The group gathered their things and walked out the kitchen door.

Elizabeth noted on the way out that the kitchen looked cleaner and brighter than it had the day before, thanks to her mom.

"I'll let you decide who sits in the front and who sits in the back," Elizabeth said as she unlocked the car doors.

As she fastened her seat belt, she waited until her mother and Goldy hopped in the back seat and her father sat up front with her. She started the car and smoothly guided it out to the main highway although at a considerably slower speed than the day before.

"Do you have anything important at the office?" Parker asked. He then corrected himself. "I'm sure it's all important and special, but do you have anything expensive enough that someone would want to steal it? Maybe try to camouflage the theft with the vandalism?"

Elizabeth shook her head. "No, most of the items are things with sentimental value. Patients who gifted me with a mug, or a special pen or dried flowers. One patient brought me a stuffed bear wearing a sweatshirt of my favorite football team."

"I didn't know you liked football," C.J. said.

Elizabeth laughed. "Well, I do. As a matter of fact, I have a habit of doing some paperwork on Sundays in front of the television so I can watch a game at the same time."

"Who knew?" C.J. asked. "Parker, are you still able to get tickets?"

He was thoughtful for a moment. "I still have a few important connections. I think I can come up with something nice. I'll let you know."

"I'll look forward to it," Elizabeth said. She slowed the car as they approached the office. There were several construction trucks there.

"Watch Goldy when she gets out of the car," Elizabeth said, concerned there was broken glass on the ground.

"You'll have to do that, because she's not going to stay with us," Parker said.

Elizabeth watched the ground as they walked and was happy to see the glass was all gone. The front door had been replaced by a large sheet of plywood. Inside the lobby, the doors had been removed from their hinges and the glass near the receptionist desk had been removed. Realizing she didn't want her parents to see the warning she'd received in her office, she asked them to stay put until she checked inside. Goldy happily followed her into the office. Elizabeth was glad to see the entire wall had already been primed. It still needed paint but the primer had covered the words enough that they were not easily recognizable. She took the moment of privacy to call Jake and let him know they were there, but they were safe and had a cleaning crew in the building with them.

Elizabeth called her parents inside her office. Together they looked around the room. The workers had piled all the papers and desk items on her conference table. The books were piled on the floor in front of the bookcase.

"Oh boy, we have some work to do," Elizabeth said.

"I'm not going to touch the books until they finish painting and put the book case back against the wall."

"This looks like a lot more than simple vandalism," C.J. said. "What did they do to the wall?"

Elizabeth looked stressed and finally said, "They spray painted curse words on it."

C.J. looked at her daughter. "Are you sure this town is safe?"

"As safe as any other in the country, Mom."

Parker turned to his daughter and raised his eyebrows.

"C'mon, let's all sit at the table. If we can sort the papers, it would be very helpful. I have a lot of reports and lab results."

"I'm assuming you have a back up in the computer?" Parker asked.

"Yes, but we print out paper copies for most patients. Not everyone likes using the computer portals yet." Elizabeth frowned for a moment. "I just realized. It's a good thing I printed out those charts in the hospital. I had them with the papers in this room. I need to find those because the only other copy was mailed to you, Dad."

"That may be what they were looking for," Parker said.

"I can't imagine why. First of all, no one knew they were here. The records are still accessible through the hospital but I would have to sign all sorts of papers to get them and I'm sure Pruitt would make it difficult for me. Anyway, let's go through this stack. If anyone finds papers with the names Frank Burdette or Connie Arturo on them, put them in a special pile. Let's just put everything else in alphabetical order."

Goldy let out a large sigh and dropped her head on Elizabeth's feet. The group worked for fifteen minutes and stopped when Goldy jumped up and ran to the door. A few seconds later, they realized she was on alert when Jake appeared at the doorway. Jake looked at the dog, who stood guard, and the group in the room. Goldy looked back but didn't growl or move.

"Is it safe to come in?"

"Of course it is. Goldy, come here. Jake is okay," Elizabeth said.

Jake took a step inside and waited for Goldy to sniff his hand. When she was satisfied, she wagged her tail and Jake approached the table. "I'm amazed at how much work they've already done here, but I'm sorry you have to go through all this."

"Thanks, I'm getting a lot of help. Jake, I'd like you to meet my parents, Dr. Parker Brooks and my mom, C.J."

Parker stood and shook Jake's hand. "I only worked in the office, my wife was the mastermind behind it."

"Oh, Parker, hush up," C.J. said as she greeted Jake.

"Glad to meet you." Jake said as he flashed a smile.

"He's the lead detective on the case," Elizabeth said to her parents before she rounded on him. "Have you found anything yet?"

Jake shook his head. "I can't say I have anything to offer just yet, but we're on it."

"I hope you'll let me know when you do," Elizabeth said.

"What did your company say about the building?" Jake asked.

"They've already started repairs. My patients are being rerouted to the Main Street office for the week and then we'll be back. They'd better be installing improved security along with the repairs."

"I'm sure they will," Jake said as he looked at the table.

"We're sorting out papers as well as my personal items."

"Mind if I join you?" Jake asked with a smile. "Maybe I'll find a clue."

Elizabeth smiled. "You're welcome to give it a try. I don't think you're going to find anything too exciting, but you never know."

Jake pulled up a chair and sat next to Elizabeth. For the next hour, they sorted and alphabetized everything they found while making small talk about the weather and sports. Questions surrounding the vandalism sat purposely unanswered as they worked to restore a relaxed atmosphere.

They had just finished when Parker's stomach growled. "Hey, does the crew get a lunch break? There's labor laws you know," Parker teased.

"Of course. We can stop anytime, especially now that the papers are done. I can do the rest during the week. They still have to paint this room anyway."

"Would you like to join us for lunch, Detective?" Parker asked while watching him for a reaction.

Jake shook his head. "As much as I would like to, I can't. Thank you for the offer, but I've got a few more stops today. It looks like everything is under control here."

Jake stood and looked at Elizabeth. "Would you mind walking me out to my car?"

"Of course not," Elizabeth said as she walked toward the door. Goldy whined. Elizabeth bent to pet her head and said, "I'll be back in a few minutes." Looking at her parents, she said, "Think about what and where you'd like to eat."

As the pair made their way out of the office, Jake turned to Elizabeth. "Have you heard anything else? Any other threats or problems?"

"No, nothing. Do you think I'll receive more?"

Jake shrugged. "It's hard to tell. It depends on whether this was a message or retaliation. We're not sure yet, but if anything happens, you call me, immediately. I'm serious, any phone calls, notes, letters, anything."

"Of course, Jake. I'll contact you immediately. Have you found something I should worry about?"

"No, nothing solid, but I feel like the case is going to break soon."

They reached the sidewalk in front of where Jake had parked. Elizabeth looked into his eyes. "Okay, be safe wherever you're going. Thanks for helping with all those papers. You didn't have to do that."

"That's okay. The more time I spend in a crime scene, the more of a feel I get for the motive and perp."

"Oh," Elizabeth felt a moment of disappointment. He was simply concentrating on his case. She looked up at him. "I know this sounds funny, but do you remember my second patient, Connie Arturo?"

"Of course," Jake said, questioning her with his eyes.

"When I was with her, near the end, she told me to tell Pasquale to look behind the credenza for an envelope. She said to make sure the police got it. I have no idea what she meant, but could you tell him for her?"

Jake looked at her without speaking. He gently touched her cheek. "Sure, but you're just telling us now?"

Elizabeth didn't know what to say. Jake tried to break the silence but the moment quickly turned awkward. As Jake got into the car, he said, "I'm glad your family is with you. Stay safe."

"I will," Elizabeth said as she turned and walked back into the office.

# CHAPTER 54

Goldy ran to Elizabeth when she walked into the room, jumped up and licked Elizabeth's arm. When Elizabeth guided her back to the floor, she whined and leaned against her side.

"I don't know why she's so clingy," C.J. said. "She's not usually like this."

Elizabeth was still petting the dog. "I don't know, but she's such a nice dog. You guys are lucky to have her."

"Yes," Parker said. "Except, she seems awfully worried about you."

"There's nothing to be worried about," Elizabeth said as she stood up. "Where do you guys want to eat lunch? Maybe we should get take out and eat at the condo so we don't have to worry about Goldy."

"I agree," C.J. said.

"How about the little Italian place we went to years ago? You remember, when you first interviewed up here? I enjoyed that restaurant," Parker suggested with a hopeful smile.

"Oh, you're talking about Mario's? Yes, they have good food and I haven't been there in a long time." She looked up the menu on her smart phone and read it aloud.

After they all choose something to eat, Elizabeth called and ordered the food for pickup in fifteen minutes. She made one last attempt to organize a few things, picked up the pile of papers and locked them in the bottom drawer of her desk. To protect her belongings, she grabbed a box and put them all inside. She planned to return the next day and look through them. She could sort them back to her desk and bookcase once the painting was done and the furniture returned to it's original position.

Closing the lights in her office, the group left, waving good-bye to the cleaning crew on the way out.

They piled into the car and Elizabeth drove to Mario's. Leaving the car running, she ran inside to pick up the food. After five minutes, she returned and placed the package in the back seat with her mom.

"The food smells great," C.J. said.

"Will Goldy bother with it?" Elizabeth asked.

"No, not Goldy. She is excellently behaved."

"Okay, let's go home and eat." Elizabeth put the car in gear and headed toward home.

When they arrived, Elizabeth opened the door to the condo and they went inside. C.J. immediately set the table as Elizabeth took Goldy for a walk. Parker plated the food, and set it on the table. When Elizabeth returned, they all sat and passed the dishes as their conversation returned to the office. Parker asked whether Jake had any new information. As Elizabeth shook her head, her cell phone buzzed.

"Hello?"

"Dr. Brooks? This is the answering service. We have a call for you from Caitlyn O'Rourke. She said she wanted to speak to you regarding a surgical emergency."

"Oh, what's the number?"

The operator rattled off the number and disconnected. Elizabeth looked up. "It's Caitlyn. She must be on call for the surgical team tonight. Excuse me, but I have to call."

"Of course," Parker said. Elizabeth realized her parents understood after all the years her father held his individual practice and was available for patients.

Elizabeth walked into the living room and dialed Caitlyn. She answered on the second ring.

"Hello?"

"Caitlyn? It's Elizabeth. What's up? Why didn't you call my cell phone?"

"I'm drowning in post-op today. We caught a surgical patient from the ER. I thought you'd want to know about this one. He says he's one of your patients. He has your name on his meds at any rate."

"What's his name?"

"John Martin. Does that ring a bell?"

Elizabeth paused for a moment. Caitlyn continued, "Says his nickname is Lucky. You'd know him from that."

"Lucky? Yes, I do know him. He's a diabetic. Why is he in the ER?"

"He came in with abdominal pain. He had a CT Scan and lab. He's very anemic."

"I had blood work drawn on him not long ago. He wasn't anemic then."

Elizabeth heard some rustling before Caitlyn started speaking. "Okay, give it to me. I'm on the phone with Dr. Brooks now. I'll ask her. Give me the report. Elizabeth? Are you there?"

"Yes, Caitlyn. What's going on?

"We just got the CT back. He's got some sort of aneurysm and I think he's slowly bleeding out. I've got a couple of surgical residents here. What do you want to do?"

Elizabeth's words came out in a rush. "Start getting him prepped. I'm coming in. Have the residents place the IV and hang fluids to stabilize him. See if Joe Dillon is on call or get whoever's covering for him. I'm on my way. I'll be there in fifteen minutes. Tell Lucky to hang on."

Elizabeth hung up the phone and hurried to get her purse and keys. She raced through the kitchen. "Sorry, I have to go to the hospital. One of my patients needs emergency surgery. I was hoping this night would end differently."

Goldy was upset and barked as she pranced up and down.

"You do what you have to do. We'll clean up," Parker said as he struggled to pull Goldy away from Elizabeth.

"Okay, but keep all the doors and windows locked," Elizabeth said as she quickly popped through the back door and closed it firmly behind her. She didn't notice the glance her parents exchanged as she ran out. Goldy barked and jumped repeatedly on the door while Parker watched and silently shook his head.

# CHAPTER 55

Elizabeth sped toward the hospital and rapidly entered the parking lot, almost breaking through the gate. She drove into the parking deck and parked as close to the door of the surgical area as she could. She ran into the locker room, threw all of her things into a locker and practically pulled on a clean pair of scrubs as she ran.

Running through the pre-op suite, she saw Caitlyn near the desk. "Hey, how is he?"

"So far, so good. When we got the call from the emergency room, I saw you were the attending of record and I knew you'd want to know about this guy. The residents will scrub in on the case. I couldn't get Dr. Joe Dillon but one of his partners will be in there as well."

"Thank you for all you do and thanks for calling me," Elizabeth said with a genuine smile. Looking around she asked, "Where's Lucky?"

"They're wheeling him into pre-op now so you have about ten minutes to scrub and get in the OR."

"Can I look at his chart and the ER record first?"

"Sure thing," Caitlyn said as she pulled up the electronic chart.

Elizabeth carefully looked at his history, physical and his lab results. He was very anemic which was new. His chest X-ray in the ER was normal as well as his EKG. He had a CT Scan which showed an abdominal aneurysm, but Lucky had no history of vascular problems. Last, she turned to his med list. It had been generated by one of the EMT's who had transported Lucky from his house. The EMT had written down the name of each pill bottle on Lucky's kitchen table.

Elizabeth scrolled down the list and stopped when she saw the supplement, MemorHold. "I don't believe it. He promised me he wasn't taking that pill."

Looking over her shoulder, Caitlyn said, "What are you looking at?"

"Lucky was taking MemorHold. He asked me several times and I told him not to start it until we got his sugar under control. Apparently, he was taking the drug anyway."

"That's the supplement you were talking about," Caitlyn said.

"Yes, the same one I reported to the FDA Safety Portal. I swear, the minute I can, I'm going to add this case to my evidence list. I'm furious. This is a bad supplement and that CEO needs to be held accountable."

The women turned when they heard a noise and watched as the transporter wheeled Lucky into pre-op. Elizabeth quickly went to his side as they locked his gurney in place.

She reached over and took his hand in hers. It was clammy and he looked very drawn and pale, as if all the air had gone out of him in the last two weeks. "Lucky, can you hear me?"

He slowly turned his head to the side. His voice was weak when he spoke. "Hey, Doc. How are you? Thanks for coming. I think I'm on my way to meet the guys from my unit. I can't complain, I got all my parts."

Elizabeth squeezed his hand. "If I have my way, you're not going anywhere. First, I'm going to make you better, then I'm going to get on you for taking those damn supplements."

Lucky gave a weak smile. "I'm sorry, Doc. I just wanted to make sure I kept my marbles and if it could help in any way, I wanted to try. I didn't think it could hurt."

Elizabeth looked up and saw the vascular surgeon enter the pre-op area. "We'll talk about it later when you get to post-op. Take it easy and have sweet dreams until then."

Lucky smiled and gave her a weak squeeze. "Don't let them forget us, Doc. Don't let them forget the veterans."

Elizabeth's stomach contracted as she felt herself getting upset. She watched as the anesthesiologist wheeled him toward the operating suite and turned to scrub. "Damn!"

"Hey, what's that all about?"

She looked up at the vascular surgeon and told him about Lucky. "He's a decent guy. He took a new supplement called MemorHold and I'm convinced it's caused this aneurysm. I told him not to take the supplement and he told me he wasn't but he was lying."

"MemorHold? Is that why we've been so busy lately?"

"I think so and if I have it my way, the FDA is going to give that company it's own colonoscopy."

"Very interesting. I'd like to spend some time talking about this tomorrow. We've had some major concerns about the number of people we've seen in surgery lately. Perhaps, this will be our answer."

"You bet, I'd be glad to," Elizabeth said as the scrub nurse helped to properly glove and gown the two doctors. When they approached the table, the residents and Lucky were ready and waiting.

The team spent the next three hours working to save Lucky's life. He was stabilized with fluids, his abdomen opened, and his aneurysm was identified and isolated. The vascular surgeon expertly removed the pathologic section of vessel and was able to properly insert a venous graft.

Checking that he was stable, the team began to close. It was a good surgical team, everyone cooperative and working together. Elizabeth relaxed a bit when she realized they had passed the most dangerous part of surgery and Lucky was still with them.

The procedure complete, he was wheeled to post-op as the team changed from their gowns and scrubs back to street dress.

Outside the locker room, Elizabeth met the vascular surgeon once again. "Will you write the orders?"

"Absolutely, I'll take the lead on this," he said. "I just saw him and he's out cold. He's not going to come out of the anesthesia for awhile."

"Okay, I appreciate the update."

"You're welcome. I know it's late on Sunday so I'll let you go, but I still want to speak with you in the hospital tomorrow about that supplement."

"That's a promise. I've had enough of this company and they have to be stopped."

"Great, well tomorrow then." He turned and headed out the door. "Have a good night."

"You too, and thanks so much for coming in," Elizabeth said as she gathered her things.

She quickly ran by the post-op suite and looked at Lucky. He was still sound asleep and looked very pale but his vitals were stable on the monitors. Elizabeth said a quick prayer that he would be okay.

Turning, she walked out of post-op, down the hall and out the door to the parking lot. She pulled her phone from her purse and as she expected, she saw that her father had called several times for updates. She hit call back and waited for him to answer as she walked to her car.

Elizabeth wasn't parked in her usual spot. She didn't have time to look for a spot under a light as she pulled into the deck. She continued to wait until her dad picked up the phone.

As she walked, she felt the hair on the back of her neck rise, her shoulders tingled. Elizabeth looked behind her and didn't see anyone or anything strange and chastised herself for being paranoid.

"Elizabeth? Elizabeth?" Parker's voice sounded from the phone but she held it near her side so she didn't hear him.

Continuing to her car, she wasn't sure if she heard footsteps behind her but again, no one was around.

Elizabeth stopped, planning to fish her keys out of her purse when she felt a hand cover her mouth. Her head was jerked backward and she dropped her purse and phone on the ground.

Her hands flailed and she was able to scratch her assailant. He yelled and slammed her against a parked car. As they struggled, a black SUV pulled up to their side. Elizabeth screamed for help, hoping someone would call 911, but when the back door of the SUV flew open and she was pushed inside she realized they were working together.

"Shut up and get in, bitch." Rough hands pushed her into the SUV and she tripped and hit her knee on the floor of the door frame. Someone pushed her forward, jumped in the SUV, and slammed the door as the car pulled away with a squeal.

"What do you want?" Elizabeth screamed from the floor.

"How about shutting up?" A man roared at her.

She tried to sit up, but was pushed down. The man sitting in the back seat moved his foot to the top of her chest and forced her to the floor. She grabbed his ankle and struggled to move it from her chest. The more she pushed the more pressure he exerted. She became short of breath and stopped struggling with him.

Elizabeth stayed still and tried to take a deep breath while looking at her captor. She was shocked to realize he was the same man from the park that Goldy went after. She must have sensed he was a danger. At that time, he hid in his car. Was he following her all day?

Holding his ankle with her hands, she tried again. "What the hell do you want?"

"I don't want anything. Just keep your mouth shut and this will be over soon. You're lucky I was told to keep you alive."

"By whom?" Elizabeth panted as his heel dug into her ribs. She couldn't move, roll over or change her position. She felt pain in her back as it twisted on the floor of the SUV. Her head dropped back to the floor of the car. She could feel the vibrations of the road on her back as the car flew through the streets.

Initially, she hadn't paid attention to the turns the driver was making and now it was too late. She couldn't trace their route without a reference point. She had no choice but to stop struggling and hope she had an opportunity to escape when the car stopped.

Elizabeth tried to look out the back window as they drove, but was unable to recognize anything in the darkness of night. She heard the driver ask a question.

"Where are we delivering to?"

"Bring her around back."

Elizabeth's stomach knotted as the car slowed down. She couldn't tell how long they had been driving, maybe ten to twenty minutes? They had to be near the hospital. Her mind raced as she tried to figure out what to do when the door opened. She was starting to panic and felt short of breath.

Elizabeth was jostled when the SUV came to a sudden stop. She heard the engine go off and the driver's door open. When the back door opened she was ready to thrust her feet forward and if she was lucky, she'd catch whomever in the sweet spot. Hopefully, she'd have enough time to run and hide.

Hearing the back door handle click, Elizabeth drew in a sharp breath. She was surprised when the rear passenger door opened and heavy hands pulled her out by her shoulders. The first goon pulled his boot off her chest to allow the driver to slide her out. She started struggling as a heavy arm held her across her chest and lifted her off her feet. She kicked as hard as she could, hoping he would let go. Her fists hit his arm in a pitiful attempt to break free.

Without thinking, she drove her elbow backward into his neck. The man yelled out, dropped her and stumbled back a step or two. His partner grabbed her by the hair, pulled her upward and slapped her on the side of her head with the back of his hand.

Elizabeth screamed and suddenly saw stars. Nausea threatened to erupt into vomiting as dizziness set in. She was pulled through a door into a dark cold room and thrown onto the floor, her head hitting concrete.

"Stupid bitch. Don't move."

Elizabeth rolled onto her side in the dark room and clutched her stomach. Her cheek was against the cold floor. Her eyes were clear when a different door opened and the silhouette of a man filled the doorframe.

# CHAPTER 56

"Elizabeth? Elizabeth? Answer me," Parker screamed into the phone. Goldy barked and ran to the kitchen door. He jumped and continued to bark as C.J. came running into the living room.

"Parker? What's going on?" His face was ashen.

"I don't know. Elizabeth called me, but never answered when I called out to her. I heard some scuffling and banging and then it sounded like tires squealing." He grabbed his wife's arm. "I think she was calling for help."

C.J.'s face looked stricken as she watched her husband.

"I don't like the sound of this. We need to call 911." His hand shook as he tried to punch the numbers on his cell phone. He turned to his wife. "What was the last name of that detective at the office today. Jake what?"

"Wagner, I think. I'm sure she said, Jake Wagner." C.J.'s voice wavered as she cried.

Parker heard a female voice on the other side of the phone. "911, what's your emergency?"

He rushed his words trying to explain something bad had happened to his daughter.

## CHAPTER 57

Elizabeth watched the silhouette fill the door frame. She noticed another man standing behind him.

"I've had enough," the silhouette yelled. She assumed it was Phil Harry. "I'm sick and tired of this and it's going to end, right now."

"Like hell it will," Elizabeth screamed. "You've got a lot more trouble coming at you."

The man in the hall yelled out. "Shut up or things will end faster than you think."

Phil Harry lurched at the doorway and the door closed. The room was completely dark and Elizabeth couldn't figure out if she was alone or if someone else was in the room. She didn't cry out for fear of sounding weak, frail or afraid. Perhaps they were purposely testing her.

A few minutes later, she heard a noise along the wall. Elizabeth realized someone else was in the room, waiting for her to move, speak, or reveal her exact location. She was glad she remained silent and now pushed herself up onto her knees. Moving slowly to the side, she wanted to distance herself from the spot she'd been in when the man entered the room. Just in case he swung a board or shot a gun in the general direction. She couldn't figure out why the lights weren't on. She was quite sure the other man in the room was Phil Harry. What kind of game was he playing?

She jumped when his voice rang out. "Where are you?"

Elizabeth kept silent and slid along the floor. She wasn't sure how far away the wall was, but she'd keep going as long as she could.

"We have to talk. It's Phil Harry. If you want to live, you'd better tell me where you are. You have no idea what's coming."

Silence. The concrete floor was cold and it felt dirty under her hands. She had no idea what dirt, bugs, or toxins could be lying there. She had no choice. It was pitch dark and smelled.

Elizabeth heard something hit the wall, followed by a crash to the floor. Phil Harry started cursing. "I don't know where you are, but you'd better start talking soon. Time is running short and there's no way this is going to end well."

She sure as hell wasn't going to help him out. Her back was against the wall and she continued sliding to the side. An irregularity in the wall alerted her to the fact that she was near a door. Trying to be as quiet as possible, she reached up for the door handle and then slowly pulled herself up to a standing position. Waiting a few seconds, she wanted to see if Phil had heard her moving. Her palm felt sweaty as her hand gripped the metal door handle.

Taking a deep breath, she pulled as hard as she could and the door opened. Light entered the room and she saw Phil Harry standing in the opposite corner, shielding his eyes with his hand. Elizabeth realized they were in a storeroom. He quickly lunged toward her. Turning, she almost fell out of the room into the hallway. She hobbled down the corridor as fast as she could go as the door slammed behind her. Turning the corner, she ran right into the chest of one of the goons who had originally thrown her into the room.

"What the hell are you doing out here?" He growled as he grabbed her by the arm. "Let's go. Since you're so full of energy, we're going to have ourselves a little party."

Elizabeth screamed and kicked as hard as she could. He picked her up as if she weighed no more than ten pounds and headed back to the room with the concrete floor. He kicked the door open while she struggled in his grasp. Yelling to the other goon, he said, "Can you put the freaking lights on and come in here and help me out?"

Elizabeth realized she was now on her stomach in the back room with the three men.

She was pushed to the floor and her arms were yanked back behind her. Before she could move, she felt something slipped over her wrists and pulled tight. She started to scream as she panicked. She felt him slap the back of her head.

"Shut up."

Elizabeth felt herself being rolled over and started to kick.

"Get off her," Phil yelled.

The goon turned around and punched Phil in the jaw. As he fell backwards, Elizabeth started to scream again. The goon grabbed her by the arms, pulled her upwards and forced her into a chair near the wall. Her eye was throbbing as the skin around the area began to swell and turn blue.

Elizabeth watched in horror and confusion as the other man put a zip tie over the hands of Phil Harry and pulled him to another chair. Looking back, he yelled to his friend. "Next time, make sure we can just off them right away. What a pain in the ass this has been, waiting for the boss."

"Shut up, he said he'll be here in a minute."

Elizabeth's head throbbed, but she realized something was drastically off. She had feared Phil Harry was going to kill her, but he was incapacitated as well. She chastised herself for not realizing there had to be darker forces in charge of the operation.

People who didn't like someone getting into their business. People who had no qualms about killing other people, especially when it wasn't by their own hand. People who didn't like losing money or being drawn into a federal limelight.

"Pay attention, he's here," the goon said as he watched the hall.

Elizabeth's eyes flicked to Phil and then to the hall as she saw a hand, holding a gun, turn the corner of the door frame. Her eyes opened in terror as she realized her blood would be spilled on the dirty concrete floor of a storeroom. She didn't want to die here, bruised and bleeding. Her face registered shock when she saw the man who entered the room.

# CHAPTER 58

Pruitt? Elizabeth shook her head. She felt confused. Pruitt was standing there, holding a gun.

"What the hell?" Elizabeth said as she watched the man before her. He walked over to where she was sitting and bent forward to look her right in the eye.

"You are the biggest pain in the ass I have ever met. Do you have any idea how much money, time and grief you've cost me?" His voice rose as his anger mounted. "The hospital was bad enough, but now that you've pulled my whole operation down, I've lost millions and millions of dollars." His neck veins pulsed, he was so enraged. "Now I have to disappear and I'll have to do it soon. If I don't, I'm looking at an FDA investigation, a surgical board review, a malpractice suit and suspension." He jabbed the barrel of the gun into her chest as he yelled. "Because of you!"

He then walked over toward Phil Harry. "And you're a worthless piece of shit. I told you to throw away all those bad samples. I told you not to let out we had a defective process but instead you let everyone take the damn stuff home until they dropped dead." He raised the gun and cold-cocked Phil Harry on the side of the head. Phil fell over and

Elizabeth grimaced at the sound of his head hitting the concrete floor of the storeroom. She yelled out to draw him away from the CEO.

"Pruitt, it was your stupid product that ruined everything. My patients wouldn't have died if they weren't on it. Your patient wouldn't have died. Your greed and massive ego did the rest. For once in your pathetic little life, man up and accept some responsibility for the stupid ass that you are."

Pruitt stood up, his face purple with rage. "That's it. You're dead."

"As if we weren't the minute your goons dragged us into this room?"

Pruitt's henchman walked up to him. "Boss, you want us to take them out and get rid of them? We probably shouldn't do anything else in here. I can get rid of the little bit of blood and hair in here but the rest we could do by the river. I know a nice little cove, no one will find nothing."

Pruitt was so pissed he was shaking. Elizabeth could tell he was paralyzed by his rage. He wanted to hurt her so bad he couldn't move, but the goon was right about leaving evidence. On the other hand, if he was leaving the country tonight, what did it matter?

Knowing she was going to die, she couldn't help herself when she shouted, "Coward. You are just a maggot and piece of garbage. Whatever life throws at you can never be bad enough to erase the true piece of crap you are."

Breaking out of his trance, Pruitt walked toward her with the gun held high. He aimed at her head and was about to pull the trigger when his body was thrust against hers and they were both knocked to the wall. The lights went off and the room was back to pitch dark.

Elizabeth's heart was pounding as she lie on her back and looked up at the ceiling. She didn't know what was happening, but she heard yelling, and screaming. A voice in the distance shouted, "Police, down on your knees." She tried to focus but her hearing became distant as the room seemed to spin around her and she lost consciousness.

A few minutes later, she awoke to find two men standing over her. One was yelling her name over and over. "Elizabeth, can you speak?

Elizabeth, look at me." She stared at the man, but couldn't seem to focus or answer his questions.

Elizabeth felt someone take her arm on the other side of her body. She turned her head and saw Jake holding her hand and smiling at her, encouraging her to focus. "Lizzie? Lizzie, can you hear me? You're going to be okay." Jake looked up at the other man. "She's going to be okay, right?"

Before she passed out once again, she heard the other man say, "Right now, let's be thankful she's alive."

# CHAPTER 59

*Elizabeth walked to the shed. The wind was calm now. The day was beautiful, sunny and warm. She felt happy, outside in the field, near the trees. She could smell the earth and freshly mowed lawn. Elizabeth turned her face toward the sun and closed her eyes as she soaked up the warmth.*

*"Beautiful place, isn't it?"*

*Elizabeth whirled around to see Frank standing beside her. She looked at him for a few minutes. For the first time, she felt calm, free and happy. The fear and anxiety were gone.*

*"I'm dead, aren't I?" Elizabeth asked as she watched his face. "It's a beautiful place to be." She looked at the trees and spied a lake behind them. The leaves rattled on their branches each time a breeze passed by. All her senses were heightened. She heard the bees and smelled the air.*

*Frank looked at her and smiled. "Elizabeth, I think we're going to be spending a lot of time together." He held out his hand and took hers. "But not now. You have so much to do and so much of your life to look forward to with those you love and those you will love."*

*Elizabeth looked up and dropped Frank's hand when she saw Connie Arturo walk toward them. Connie stood by Frank and wrapping her hand around his arm, she rested her head against him. With his other hand, Frank placed it on Connie's arm and held her close.*

*"Go back, Elizabeth. We'll be in touch when we need to be. Go live your life and appreciate every day, every hour as you do."*

*Frank turned toward Connie, kissed her on the nose and the two turned and walked toward the lake.*

ELIZABETH HEARD something beep as she felt the first stab of pain in her head. She smelled antiseptic. As she became more awake, she felt stiff as she tried to move. Someone gasped in the corner of the room.

Trying to open her eyes, Elizabeth's head felt heavy. She felt a cool hand on hers. "Elizabeth, honey, are you awake?"

Elizabeth's eyelids fluttered as she turned toward the voice. She saw her parents standing by the side of the bed. Parker smiled and grabbed her hand as her mother choked up. Behind them, she saw an attractive man in a beautiful suit. Jake stood up and smiled at her.

Parker leaned toward her. "You're safe now, Lizzie. You just need some time to heal."

# CHAPTER 60

Three days later, Jake pushed her wheelchair down the hall of the hospital. "Where are we going?" Elizabeth asked as they proceeded forward.

"We're going to a special room so we can talk."

"Why can't we talk in my room?"

"Because it's time for you to get up and out. We can't have you getting used to too much relaxation."

"I knew it wouldn't last," Elizabeth said as she sighed deeply.

"As a matter of fact, you're going home in a few days, so you should get used to it."

"I know, my mom and dad have already made arrangements to pick me up," Elizabeth said with a shrug.

"They've been very worried about you," Jake said as he turned the corner of the hall and headed for the solarium.

As they approached the room, Elizabeth heard some commotion. When she looked inside she saw Caitlyn, Heather, her parents and Goldy. There was a cake on the table and balloons around the room.

Goldy pulled free from Parker as soon as she was in view and leapt toward the wheelchair.

The crowd laughed and cheered as the dog placed her front paws on Elizabeth's lap, stretched up and licked her face. "Goldy, Goldy, how are you girl?"

"She's been crazy. We had to bring her in to see you. I've never seen such an agitated dog as this one. She's been miserable from the minute you left to do Lucky's surgery."

Elizabeth looked up at Caitlyn and Heather. "How is Lucky?"

"He's doing well," Caitlyn said. "Dr. Dillon is taking care of him, but he's been asking to see you. He wants us to wheel him down to your room, but we haven't done it yet. We wanted to wait until you're ready."

"Did Dr. Dillon say he'll have a full recovery?"

"Apparently so," Caitlyn said. "Lucky wants to beg your forgiveness for taking the supplement when you told him not to."

Shaking her head, Elizabeth grinned. "At least he's here to do so."

She turned to Heather. "How's the office?"

"It's beautiful. They painted and cleaned everything and we got all new furniture. We moved back yesterday. Your office is good as new. I think I put everything in the right place but you can fix it when you come back."

"Who wants a piece of cake?" C.J. called from across the room. The group gathered near the table and C.J. passed out paper plates with slices of cake on each one with a plastic fork.

Elizabeth took a plate and tasted the delicious cake. Much better than hospital food. Goldy stayed at her side, leaning against Elizabeth's legs. Elizabeth put her plate down so she could continue to pet the dog's head.

"That was delicious and as much as I would love to stay, I have to go back to my shift." Caitlyn threw the plate in the garbage and gave her friend a hug around the shoulders. "I can't wait for you to come back. You cannot believe all the drama in the hospital now that Pruitt is gone. The staff and the gossip have gone wild. The hospital has started the search for a new Chief of Surgery but in the meantime they talked Dr. Bruce Covington into taking the interim position. It's wild."

Elizabeth's eyes opened wide. "Oh boy. That must be something.

Dr. Covington is wonderful. I can't wait to hear what they're saying about me."

"Let's just say there are some interesting theories. Come back to work soon so I can tell you all about it."

"Yes, I agree," Heather said as she gave her a hug as well. The two women turned and left the room.

"They're such great friends," Elizabeth said as she watched them go. Elizabeth turned the wheelchair toward the table. She looked at her parents and Jake sitting together. Goldy was at her side.

"Okay, now that it's just us, I want the truth. It's been a couple of days and I want to be told everything." Elizabeth looked at her dad. "I know you've spoken to my physician several times and you've looked over the MRI. What's the verdict, Doc?"

Parker shrugged. "Everything looks good. Your brain looks completely normal on exam. No fractures, no bleeds, no tumors, nothing to worry about."

"And my lab?"

"Also normal," Parker smiled.

"No need for a psych eval?"

"I can't find a reason you would need one. As soon as your headaches go away from the concussion, you should be fine."

Parker's voice softened when he asked her, "Have you been having any dreams?"

She looked up at him and said, "Not a one."

Elizabeth gave her parents a pointed look before she turned to look at Jake. "Okay, it's your turn. I want to know what happened after I passed out in that room."

"Well, I guess you deserve to know that," Jake said. "Although, I want to hear exactly what you remember. I'll back up a bit to let you know what we've surmised so far. After you finished in surgery, you were on your way out to your car and tried to call your father. He picked up the phone and was listening to you walking to your car, but I guess you were already distracted. He heard the men when they abducted you, heard you cry out, but then heard nothing. He immediately called 911 and asked them to track me down."

Elizabeth nodded. "I remember I was in the back of a SUV, on the floor, and the big goon had his foot on top of me so I couldn't move. We drove for awhile until we got to that dirty storeroom."

"Yes, the storeroom was in a building in the very back of the MemorHold property."

"That makes sense," Elizabeth said. "Phil Harry came in to the storeroom and was screaming he'd had enough. I started screaming back, because I thought he was yelling at me. That's the funny part. Apparently, he was yelling at the goons who forced him into the room. When they threw him in there, the lights were off and the room was pitch black. I was confused because I thought he was trying to kill me so I slowly crawled along the storeroom wall until I got to the door. I managed to stand up and open it but I ran right into the driver who dragged me back to the room. Thats when they tied our hands and forced us to sit while we waited for the boss. I can't tell you how shocked I was when Pruitt walked into the room, holding a gun."

"Total ass that he is," Jake said. "Then what happened."

Elizabeth began to shake. "Pruitt was enraged. He was screaming and turning purple. He wanted to hurt me so bad. My head got knocked around enough against the concrete floor, but he wanted to kill me right there. He was furious about me calling the federal government."

"That's the funny thing, the FDA hadn't responded yet." Parker explained.

"I told him. When he yelled at me in the café that day, I told him I called the FDA and he went nuts. I thought he was mad that they would come to the hospital and look into the deaths. I had no idea he was the mastermind. He must have started planning my demise from that very minute on. But he was also angry with Phil Harry. It sounded like he hired him as an empty suit, but Phil didn't listen to all the orders he'd been given which is why Pruitt blamed him. He used the gun and cold-cocked him right on the side of the head. His head cracked against the floor." Elizabeth looked at Jake and her father. "How is he?"

Parker was quiet as Jake looked back at him and nodded. "He has a concussion, but he's getting better. On the bright side, he looked much worse than you."

"Dad," Elizabeth said although with a smile.

Jake broke in. "He's singing like a canary. He's given us quite a bit of useful information about Pruitt and MemorHold. He desperately wants to keep himself out of jail."

"I still don't understand what happened to Pruitt in the end. He was just about to kill us right there and then, but his goons were trying to hold him off until they could bring us near the river and dump our bodies."

C.J. got upset and walked to the other side of the room as Elizabeth watched her go.

Jake cleared his throat. "That's where we came in. We blew the door. Pruitt was standing in front of you and the blast threw him into you and thrust both of you into the wall. He was knocked out cold. He tried to claim he had back pain but he's resting comfortably in a jail cell right now."

"I hope he's not too comfortable," Elizabeth said, getting upset.

"No, believe me, he's not. He's got all the alphabet agencies lining up to see him. DEA, FBI, DOJ, you name it. He'll be in jail for quite a while in addition to losing his license, and being sued for malpractice and everyone he's screwed with this company. Your first patient that died, Frank Burdette, was the accountant. Pruitt was taking money off the top and trying to set Frank up for embezzlement. Pruitt had set him up quite nicely but his plan was ruined when Frank accidentally died after surgery. That's the real reason he was angry, not because of your technique, but because you messed up his money flow."

"Greedy, arrogant, bastard," Elizabeth said as she shook her head. "What about Connie? Was he trying to blame her too?"

"No, she was just trying to help Frank. They were good friends."

Elizabeth looked at Jake. "What about the envelope? Did Pasquale find it?"

Jake smiled. "Yes, he did and he gave it to us."

"What was in it?"

"Account ledgers. It appears Frank was on to Pruitt's plan so he copied all the ledgers and checks and gave them to Connie to hold in case anything happened to him. Before surgery, he had a conversation with officials and had promised to help them. He made a deal so that he wouldn't be prosecuted and figured he would be safe in the hospital in the meantime."

"What about Connie and Pasquale?"

"She was trying to help Frank get out. Pasquale cried when he realized she died from taking the supplements. She brought them home for both of them but he didn't take them. He was worried she was having an affair with Frank. Pasquale loved her very much."

"And I think she still loved him," Elizabeth said. "She wanted him to know she never stopped loving him and was always faithful."

Elizabeth paused for a moment and teared up when she looked at her family and Jake. "I hope everything else turns out okay."

"It will," Parker said. "The lawsuit against you has already been dropped. The surgical department is no longer investigating your surgical skill and your staff and patients miss you terribly."

Elizabeth reached out and squeezed their hands. "Thank you for being there and for saving my life."

Parker placed his hand on his daughter's shoulder. "Goldy was trying to tell us all along. She went nuts when you left the house and wouldn't stop. When I heard you scream over the phone and lost contact, I had to call 911 and Jake right away."

Elizabeth thought for a moment and looked at them. "How did you know where to find me? Lucky guess?"

"You know, It's a good thing you sent me that text, otherwise I don't think you would have been lucky. Between that and your father, I was able to track your phone."

"What text?" Elizabeth asked, confused.

"I guess you were able to get off a quick text before you were grabbed. You probably don't remember with your concussion," Jake said. "Here I saved it for evidence." Jake punched a few things on his phone and showed Elizabeth.

*Please Help me*
*With Phil Harry*
*Gonna kill me*
*FB*

"AT THE END, I guess you were just hitting random buttons."

Elizabeth looked at the text and froze. She knew she hadn't texted anyone before her cell phone dropped to the parking deck floor and she didn't know about Phil until she got to the storeroom. FB? Frank Burdette. "You found my phone in the parking deck, right?"

"Yeah, and when I read this, I called Harry's administrative assistant and insisted she give me his cell phone number. He must have been in the SUV when they grabbed you. I found you by tracking the location of his phone. Thankfully, it worked, but please don't ever do anything like that again. I don't think I could take it," Jake said as he leaned forward, kissed her cheek and hugged her as her mom raised her eyebrows and smiled at Parker.

Elizabeth blushed and hugged him back. She remained thoughtful and silently offered her thanks to Frank for saving her life. Seeing her parents behind Jake's back she smiled at them in anticipation of nothing more than sweet dreams in her future.

# ABOUT THE AUTHOR

Linda Rawlins is an American writer of mystery fiction best known for her Misty Point Mystery Series. She is also the author of the Rocky Meadow Mysteries including The Bench, Fatal Breach and Sacred Gold. She loved to read as a child and started writing her first mystery novel in fifth grade. She then went on to study science, medicine and literature, eventually graduating medical school and establishing her career in medicine.

Linda Rawlins lives in New Jersey with her husband, her family and spoiled dog. She loves spending time at the beach as well as visiting the mountains of Vermont. She is an active member of Mystery Writers of America as well as the 2018 Central Jersey VP of Sisters in Crime.

Visit Linda at lindarawlins.com and sign up for her mailing list to be the first to know about new releases, appearances, and more.

facebook.com/lindarawlinsauthor

twitter.com/lrl8

instagram.com/lindarawlins

## ALSO BY LINDA RAWLINS

The Misty Point Mystery Series

Misty Manor

Misty Point

Misty Winter

Misty Treasure

The Rocky Meadow Mystery Series

The Bench

Fatal Breach

Sacred Gold

Made in the USA
Monee, IL
08 November 2026

67994723R00163